AF333478

Topics in Neuroscience

Managing Editor:

GIANCARLO COMI

Co-Editor:

JACOPO MELDOLESI

Associate Editors:

MASSIMO FILIPPI

LETIZIA LEOCANI

GIANVITO MARTINO

Springer

Milano
Berlin
Heidelberg
New York
Hong Kong
London
Paris
Tokyo

O.R. Hommes • G. Comi (Eds)

Early Indicators
Early Treatments
Neuroprotection
in Multiple Sclerosis

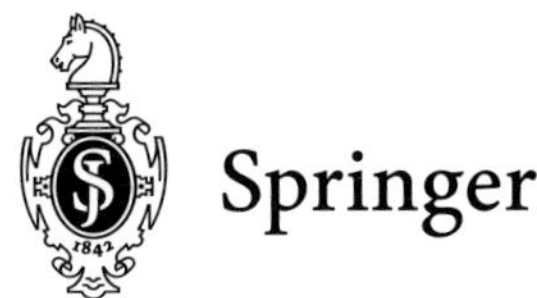

Springer

OTTO R. HOMMES
European Charcot
Foundation
Nijmegen, The Netherlands

GIANCARLO COMI
Department of Neurology
Scientific Institute and University
Ospedale San Raffaele, Milan, Italy

The Editors and Authors wish to thank SCHERING S.p.A. for the support and help in the realization and promotion of this volume

---

Springer-Verlag is a part of Springer Science+Business Media

springeronline.com

ISBN 88-470-0195-1

Library of Congress Cataloging-in-Publication Data:
Early indicators, early treatment, neuroprotection in multiple sclerosis / O. Hommes, G. Comi.
    p. cm. – (Topics in neuroscience)
  Includes bibliographical references and index.
  ISBN 8847001951 (alk. paper)
  1. Multiple sclerosis – Pathophysiology. 2. Multiple sclerosis – Treatment. I. Hommes, Otto R.
  (Otto Roelf) II. Comi, G. (Giancarlo), 1947 – III. Series.

  RC377.E27 2003
  616.8'34-dc22

                                                                    2003065478

Typesetting: Color Point Srl (Milan)
Printing and binding: Staroffset (Cernusco sul Naviglio, Milan)
Cover design: Simona Colombo

Printed in Italy

SPIN: 10970409

Foreword

There is now evidence that irreversible brain damage accumulates very early in the course of multiple sclerosis. This book reviews the main neurobiological, magnetic resonance imaging, and clinical aspects of the early phases of the disease. Mechanisms of irreversible axonal damage and the role played by the interaction of glia and the axon are highlighted.

In contrast to what was believed for a long time, the sufficient availability of oligodendrocyte precursor cells to promote remyelination in acute lesions has now been demonstrated. For reasons not understood, this remyelination process fails or does not start, particularly in the chronic stages of the disease.

These findings emphasize the importance of the "milieu" changes induced by an inflammatory process in limiting remyelination. However, first indications are that part of this inflammatory process may have a neuroprotective effect.

Pathological studies in multiple sclerosis have now clearly demonstrated that destructive processes may be followed by recovery phases in such a way that myelin may be morphologically and functionally reconstituted.

These findings provide the rationale for early treatment and emphasize the importance of clinical trials in early multiple sclerosis. Early treatment is one of the most important aspects in multiple sclerosis today.

Milan, October 2003

O.R. Hommes
G. Comi

Table of Contents

List of Contributors

A. Achiron
Multiple Sclerosis Center,
Sheba Medical Center,
Tel-Hashomer, Israel

S. Amor
Department of Immunobiology, BPRC,
Rijswijk, The Netherlands

F. Bagnato
Department of Neurological Sciences,
University "La Sapienza",
Rome, Italy

Y. Barak
Multiple Sclerosis Center,
Sheba Medical Center,
Tel-Hashomer, Israel

F. Barkhof
Department of Radiology,
VU Medical Center,
Amsterdam, The Netherlands

T. Berger
Department of Neurology,
University of Innsbruck,
Innsbruck, Austria

L. Bergers
Department of Radiology,
VU Medical Center,
Amsterdam, The Netherlands

C. Bjartmar
Department of Neurosciences,
Lerner Research Institute,
Cleveland Clinic Foundation,
Cleveland, USA

L. Bozzao
Department of Neurological Sciences,
University "La Sapienza",
Rome, Italy

E.C.W. Breij
Department of Molecular Cell Biology
and Immunology, VU Medical Centre,
Amsterdam, The Netherlands

A. Capurso
Department of Geriatrics,
Center for Aging Brain, Memory Unit,
University of Bari, Policlinico,
Bari, Italy

C. Capurso
Department of Geriatrics,
Center for Aging Brain, Memory Unit,
University of Bari, Policlinico,
Bari, Italy

S. Capurso
Department of Geriatrics,
Center for Aging Brain, Memory Unit,
University of Bari, Policlinico,
Bari, Italy

F. Caramia
Department of Neurological Sciences,
University "La Sapienza",
Rome, Italy

M. Cohen
Multiple Sclerosis Center,
Sheba Medical Center,
Tel-Hashomer, Israel

I.R. Cohen
Department of Immunology,
Weizmann Institut of Science,
Rehovot, Israel
e-mail: Irun.Cohen@Weizmann.ac.il

A.M. Colacicco
Department of Geriatrics,
Center for Aging Brain, Memory Unit,
University of Bari, Policlinico,
Bari, Italy

A.J. Coles
University of Cambridge Neurology
Unit, Addenbrooke's Hospital,
Cambridge, UK

G. Comi
Multiple Sclerosis Centre,
Department of Neurology,
Scientific Institute and University,
Ospedale San Raffaele,
Milan, Italy

A. Compston
University of Cambridge Neurology
Unit, Addenbrooke's Hospital;
MCR Cambridge, Centre for Brain Repair,
Cambridge, UK

C.M. Davie
NMR Research Unit,
Institute of Neurology,
London, UK

F. Deisenhammer
Department of Neurology,
University of Innsbruck,
Innsbruck, Austria

J. De Keyser
Department of Neurology,
Academisch Ziekenhuis Groningen,
Groningen, The Netherlands

N. De Stefano
Neurometabolic Unit,
Institute of Neurological Sciences,
University of Siena, Siena, Italy

C.D. Dijkstra
Department of Molecular Cell Biology
and Immunology,
VU Medical Centre,
Amsterdam, The Netherlands

S. Di Legge
Department of Neurological Sciences,
University "La Sapienza",
Rome, Italy

E. Dilitz
Department of Neurology,
University of Innsbruck,
Innsbruck, Austria

A. D'Introno
Department of Geriatrics,
Center for Aging Brain, Memory Unit,
University of Bari, Policlinico,
Bari, Italy

R. Egg
Department of Neurology,
University of Innsbruck,
Innsbruck, Austria

M. Faibel
Multiple Sclerosis Center,
Sheba Medical Center,
Tel-Hashomer, Israel

M. Filippi
Neuroimaging Research Unit,
Department of Neuroscience,
Scientific Institute and University
Ospedale San Raffaele, Milan, Italy

G. Giovannoni
Departments of Neurochemistry
and Clinical Neurology,
Institute of Neurology,
London, UK

R.E. Gonsette
National Center for MS,
Melsbroek, Belgium

G. Hale
Therapeutic Antibody Centre,
Headington, Oxford;
Sir William Dunn School of Pathology,
Oxford, UK

C.E. Hayes
Department of Biochemistry, University
of Wisconsin-Madison, Madison,
WI, USA

K. Hoekstra
Department of Molecular Cell Biology
and Immunology,
VU Medical Centre,
Amsterdam, The Netherlands

V. Hummel
Clinical Research Unit for Multiple
Sclerosis and Neuroimmunology,
University of Würzburg,
Würzburg, Germany

L. Jacobs
Department of Radiology/MRI
University of Colorado Health Sciences
Center, Denver, CO, USA

P.J.H. Jongen
Multiple Sclerosis Centre, Nijmegen,
The Netherlands

N. Kalkers
Department of Neurology,
VU Medical Center,
Amsterdam, The Netherlands

B.A. Kallmann
Clinical Research Unit for Multiple
Sclerosis and Neuroimmunology, Julius-
Maximilians-Universität,
Würzburg, Germany

D.I. Kaufman
Department of Neurology and
Ophthalmology, Michigan State University
East Lansing, MI, USA

I. Kishner
Multiple Sclerosis Center,
Sheba Medical Center,
Tel-Hashomer, Israel

M. Kortekaas
Department of Molecular Cell Biology
and Immunology,
VU Medical Centre,
Amsterdam, The Netherlands

G.L. Lenzi
Department of Neurological Sciences,
University "La Sapienza",
Rome, Italy

O. Lidman
Neuroimmunology Unit,
Department of Medicine,
Karolinska Institute, Karolinska Hospital,
Stockholm, Sweden

C. Linington
Department of Neuroimmunology,
Max-Planck-Institut for Neurobiology,
Martinsried, Germany

D. Miller
NMR Research Unit,
Institute of Neurology
London, UK

A. Minagar
MS Center, Department of Neurology,
University of Miami School of Medicine
Miami, FL, USA

S. Miron
Multiple Sclerosis Center,
Sheba Medical Center,
Tel-Hashomer, Israel

L. Moiola
Multiple Sclerosis Centre,
Department of Neurology,
Scientific Institute and University
Ospedale San Raffaele,
Milan, Italy

P. Molyneux
NMR Research Unit,
Institute of Neurology,
London, UK

W. Nucciarelli
Department of Neurological Sciences,
University "La Sapienza",
Rome, Italy

T. Olsson
Neuroimmunology Unit,
Department of Medicine,
Karolinska Institute, Karolinska Hospital,
Stockholm, Sweden

P. Pantano
Department of Neurological Sciences,
University "La Sapienza",
Rome, Italy

F. Panza
Department of Geriatrics,
Center for Aging Brain, Memory Unit,
University of Bari, Policlinico,
Bari, Italy

A. Paolillo
NMR Research Unit,
Institute of Neurology
London, UK;
Department of Neurological Sciences,
University "La Sapienza",
Rome, Italy

M.C. Piattella
Department of Experimental Medicine,
University "La Sapienza",
Rome, Italy

F. Piehl
Neuroimmunology Unit,
Department of Medicine,
Karolinska Institute, Karolinska Hospital,
Stockholm, Sweden

Ch. Polman
Department of Neurology,
VU Medical Center,
Amsterdam, The Netherlands

C. Pozzilli
Department of Neurological Sciences,
University "La Sapienza",
Rome, Italy

G. Ramsaransing
Department of Neurology,
Academisch Ziekenhuis Groningen,
Groningen, The Netherlands

M. Reindl
Department of Neurology,
University of Innsbruck,
Innsbruck, Austria

P. Rieckmann
Clinical Research Unit for Multiple
Sclerosis and Neuroimmunology,
University of Würzburg,
Würzburg, Germany

P. Rubner
Department of Neurology,
University of Innsbruck,
Innsbruck, Austria

I. Sarova-Pinhas
Multiple Sclerosis Center,
Sheba Medical Center,
Tel-Hashomer, Israel

W.A. Sheremata
MS Center, Department of Neurology,
University of Miami School of Medicine
Miami, FL, USA

J.H. Simon
Department of Radiology/MRI,
University of Colorado Health Sciences
Center, Denver, CO, USA

N. Simonian
Department of Radiology/MRI,
University of Colorado Health Sciences
Center, Denver, CO, USA

V. Solfrizzi
Department of Geriatrics,
Center for Aging Brain, Memory Unit,
University of Bari, Policlinico,
Bari, Italy

D. Stadlbauer
Department of Neurology,
University of Innsbruck,
Innsbruck, Austria

Y. Stern
Multiple Sclerosis Center,
Sheba Medical Center,
Tel-Hashomer, Israel

K.V. Toyka
Clinical Research Unit for Multiple
Sclerosis and Neuroimmunology,
University of Würzburg,
Würzburg, Germany

B.D. Trapp
Department of Neurosciences,
Lerner Research Institute,
Cleveland Clinic Foundation,
Cleveland, USA

A. van der Goes
Department of Molecular Cell Biology
and Immunology,
VU Medical Centre,
Amsterdam, The Netherlands

R. van Schijndel
Department of Clinical Physics
and Informatics,
VU Medical Center,
Amsterdam, The Netherlands

H. Waldmann
Sir William Dunn School of Pathology,
Oxford, UK

N. Wilczak
Department of Neurology,
Academisch Ziekenhuis Groningen,
Groningen, The Netherlands

M.G. Wing
University of Cambridge Neurology
Unit, Addenbrooke's Hospital,
Cambridge, UK

E. Zeinstra
Department of Neurology,
Academisch Ziekenhuis Groningen,
Groningen, The Netherlands

Chapter 1

Evidence for an Early Treatment of Multiple Sclerosis

G. COMI, L. MOIOLA

Introduction

Multiple sclerosis (MS) is a disease leading to a significant disability in the vast majority of patients [1, 2]. The available immunomodulatory treatments are not a cure for MS, but there is clear evidence from class I clinical trials that they significantly reduce the disease activity and delay the increase of disability in relapsing-remitting patients [3-10]. However, the positive effects are less clear in secondary progressive patients [11, 12]. The different effects of immunomodulatory treatments according to the disease course is probably explained by the complex pathogenesis of MS. Indications on the use of available therapies for MS have substantially changed in a few years, passing from a conservative [13, 14] to a more-aggressive attitude [15]. It is interesting to note that the consensus statement of the Canadian MS Clinic Network, recently published [15], on the use of disease modifying agents in MS, requires evidence of ongoing disease activity, which can be based on clinical or magnetic resonance imaging (MRI) data. The previous consensus of treatment [13, 14, 16, 17] required two or more relapses in the last 2 years in order to start treatment. These changes are probably explained by the results of the new trials testing the efficacy and safety of interferons and glatiramer acetate [5-7, 10], by the experience acquired during these years, and by the recent knowledge of the pathophysiology of the disease. The demonstration of early irreversible axonal damage is a strong argument in favor of early treatment, an option that is beginning to be favored by many neurologists [18, 19].

Rationale for Early Treatment

Many factors, summarized in Table 1, support early treatment in MS. Some clinical and imaging findings, observed at clinical presentation of MS, are predictive

Table 1. Rationale for an early treatment of multiple sclerosis

Reduction of disease activity in the early phases (prognostic implications)
Antigen spreading
Longitudinal changes of immunopathology
Prevention of irreversible pathological changes
Evidence of a better response to immunoactive therapies in patients with:
    – less disability at treatment onset
    – younger age at treatment onset

of the evolution to clinically definite MS (CDMS) and of future disability. The most important factors are the amount of nervous tissue affected by the disease, and the presence of brain active lesions as revealed by MRI techniques [20-22]. In the study performed by Filippi et al. [20] in patients with isolated syndromes, the baseline T2 lesion load was predictive of the future disability; extension to 10 years of the same study [21] confirmed the previous results.

In the Early Treatment of Multiple Sclerosis Study (ETOMS), patients with 9 or more T2 lesions on brain MRI, had a more-frequent conversion to CDMS over 2 years than patients with 4-8 lesions (Fig. 1) [23]. Interestingly, the risk was the same in patients with 9-25 lesions and in patients with more than 25 lesions. In the same study, the presence of enhancing lesions on the baseline scan, which was performed in two-thirds of patients 2-3 months after the attack onset, suggests that the persistence of inflammatory activity is predictive of the future conversion to CDMS [23].

There are at least two possible explanations for these early prognostic factors. Some genetic factors might influence the disease evolution, for instance some patients may accumulate lesions faster than others. This interpretation is supported by the heterogeneity of MS pathogenesis [24]. Soldestrom et al. [25] in a follow-up study performed in optic neuritis (ON) patients found that the Dw2 phenotype was related to the development of MS. Sciacca et al. [26] found that a

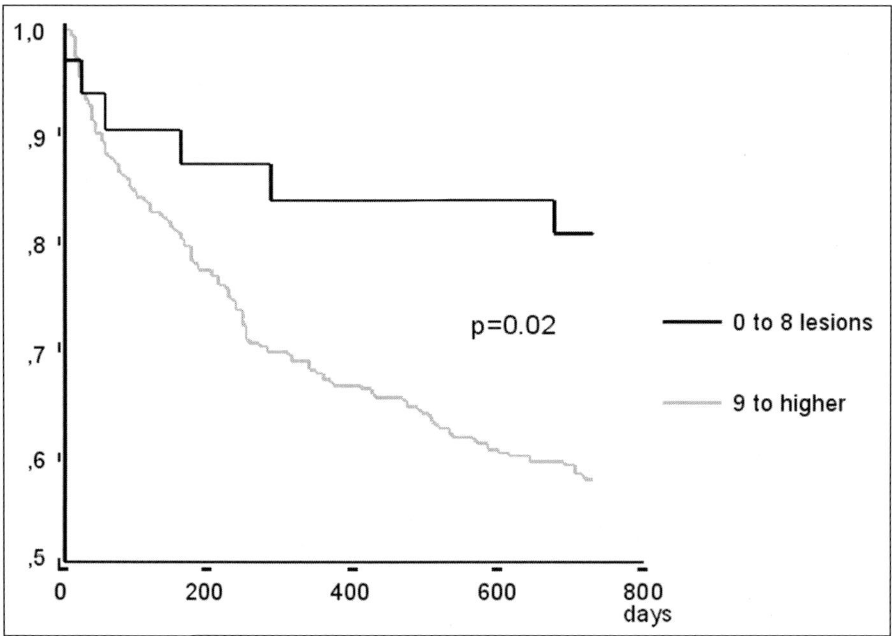

Fig. 1. Kaplan Meier lifetable analysis of the cumulative probability of clinically definite multiple sclerosis according to the number of MRI lesions

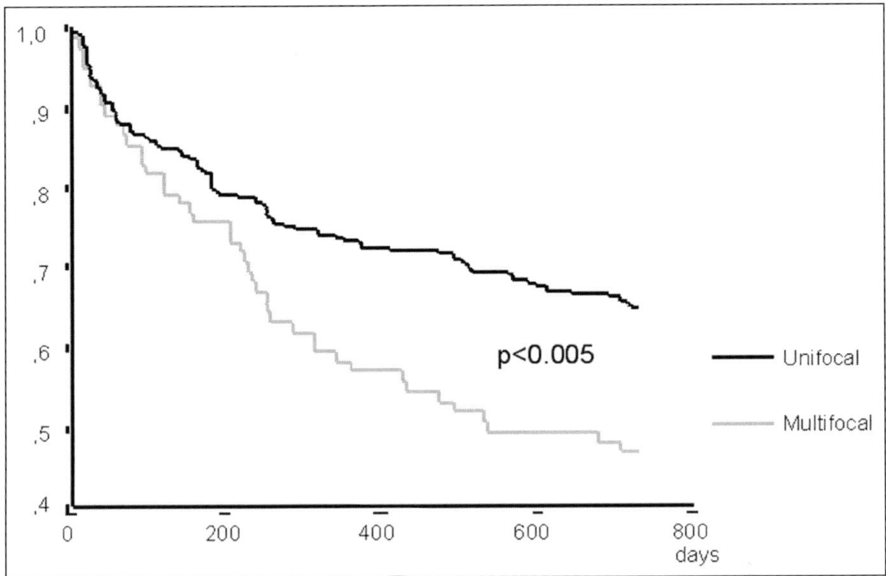

Fig. 2. Kaplan Meier lifetable analysis of the cumulative probability of clinically definite multiple sclerosis according to the unifocal or multifocal presentation

more-aggressive disease course was associated with the A1/A1 genotype of the anti-inflammatory cytokine interleukin-1 (IL-1) receptor antagonist. A second possibility is that patients with more brain MRI lesions at onset have a longer subclinical phase of the disease. However, this interpretation does not explain why patients with a multifocal rather than unifocal presentation, as indicated by clinical findings, also more frequently convert to CDMS (Fig. 2) [23]. Moreover, it is well known that a high relapse rate in the early phases of the disease and a short interval between first and second attack are related to a worse prognosis [27, 28]. If a high clinical and MRI activity in the early phases results in a more-rapid accumulation of irreversible disability, we can expect that a treatment able to reduce disease activity in the early phases may substantially ameliorate the long-term prognosis.

Immunological Findings

To date there is no definite evidence that immunological abnormalities observed in early and late phases of the disease differ significantly. However, some scattered reports support the possibility of an increased complexity over time of the immunological derangement underlying the pathogenesis of MS. In autoimmunity, regulatory cells tend to recognize more epitopes within the same antigen and more antigens within the same organ over time during the progression of the disease; this process, which is called inter-/intra-epitope spreading, is a feature of central nervous system (CNS) antigen-specific T cells from animals with experimental allergic encephalomyelitis (EAE) [29]. Mice immunized with the immunodominant proteolipid protein (PLP) 139-151 determinant had an intra- and intermolecular sequential determinant spreading. Interestingly, only mice with relapsing progressive courses had the spreading of recognition to new immunodominant encephalitogenic determinants [29]. The same group of researchers [30] also demonstrated that self recognition associated with the development of MS is a process characterized by autoreactive diversity, plasticity, and instability. However, it is not clear whether autoreactivity stabilizes with time or maintains a high level of diversity and plasticity during the disease.

Patients with progressive MS show significantly increased interferon-γ (IFN-γ) production compared with relapsing-remitting MS patients when T cells are stimulated with anti-CD3 antibody. This increased production is IL-12 dependent, and progressive MS patients show increased IL-12 production compared with relapsing-remitting MS patients [31, 32]. These data suggest that the inflammatory process may have different characteristics as the disease evolves; if these phenomena play a role in the disease evolution, an early immunomodulatory treatment leading to downregulation of antigen-specific T cells and the selective activation of specific cytokine networks could give better results than a delayed treatment and maybe halt disease progression.

Pathology and Pathophysiology

There is much converging clinical, pathological, neurophysiological, and MRI evidence that irreversible axonal damage occurs from the early phases of the disease, although the degree of damage can be quite variable from patient to patient. Pathological observations might explain the inter-patient variability of MS course. There are multiple pathological patterns in MS, probably due to variable pathogenetic mechanisms [33]. However, in the same patient, at a given time, all the lesions share the same pathological patterns [34]. Whether the same pathological pattern will be persistent throughout life is still unclear; if this is the case, then the prognosis could be determined in the early phases of the disease and specific therapeutic strategies could be adopted.

The pathological substrates symptoms and signs in MS are demyelination and axonal degeneration. Demyelination results in an instability of nerve conduction and generation of ectopic impulses, responsible for some typical positive MS symptoms, like Lhermitte sign, and negative symptoms and signs due to conduction block. Conduction block is due to segmental demyelination and the action of toxic substances, like nitricoxide and free radicals, produced by the inflammation, which can easily gain access to axons exposed by demyelination [35].

Reversible conduction block is responsible for the transitory neurological dysfunction observed in acute bouts. It is still debatable whether a persistent conduction block may also arise in the CNS, as in the peripheral nervous system, for example in the multifocal motor conduction block neuropathy. Nevertheless it is clear that the pathological basis for persistent neurological dysfunction in MS is axonal damage.

In Charcot's description in 1877 [36], the axonal pathology inside MS plaques was considered of limited importance. This view was accepted for a long time. Putman in 1936 [37] first claimed the importance of axonal pathology in MS. In a post-mortem study, he found a severe axonal loss in 50% of the plaques. In contrast, Greenfield and King [38] in the same year reported a nearly normal axonal density in most plaques. Some recent pathological studies have clearly demonstrated that axonal pathology also occurs in the early phases of the disease. The pathophysiology of axonal damage is quite complex and not fully understood. At least three different mechanisms can be hypothesized.

Failure of Remyelination

Axonal structure is modulated by myelination. The areas of axonal loss are greater in plaques and degenerated axons are not surrounded by myelin. Demyelination affects the cytoskeletal structure, which impairs axonal transport and contributes to axonal degeneration. During the early relapsing-remitting stage of disease evolution, extensive remyelination is usually observed, which explains the full recovery characterizing most of the bouts in this phase of the disease [39, 40]. Remyelination depends upon the availability of olygodendrocytes or their progenitor cells within the lesions [41, 42]. It has been suggested that the failure of myelin repair in late chronic lesions could be due to a depletion of this progenitor cell pool, which is likely to occur in areas of repeated demyelinating episodes [43]. Both pathological studies and MRI studies revealed that about 30% of the active lesions are old lesions reactivated, the so-called shadow plaques. The same findings have been clearly demonstrated in EAE. The final result is a secondary axonal degeneration leading to a permanent neurological dysfunction.

Early Axonal Damage

Ferguson et al. [44], using β-amyloid precursor protein, demonstrated the presence of damaged axons in both acute and active chronic MS lesions, i.e., in areas of acute inflammation. Trapp et al. [45] in a very elegant study utilized confocal microscopy and immunohistochemistry to demonstrate a large number of transected axons in active lesions. The frequency of terminal axonal ovoids, indicating recent axonal transection, correlated with active inflammation. Axonal damage might be a consequence of the loss of myelin exposing the axon to the insult of the products of inflammation or a humoral immune response could perhaps contribute to the irreversible axonal damage. Raine et al. [46] very recently provided evidence that antibody to myelin oligodendrocyte glycoprotein (MOG) may contribute to the myelin damage. Antibodies to MOG have been shown to be specifically bound to disintegrated myelin around axons in acute MS lesions as well as in marmoset EAE. Moreover, we cannot exclude the pathogenetic role of antibodies to axonal components.

Because of the redundancy characterizing the organization of the CNS and because of the convergency/divergency of the multi-synaptic pathways, the initial axonal loss does not produce permanent symptoms and signs. However, new lesions affecting the same pathways or reactivation of old lesions will result in a severe axonal loss and will determine irreversible neurological dysfunctions.

Secondary Axonal Degeneration

Trapp et al. [45] also found diffuse abnormalities in surviving axons, discontinuous staining of the axons, and modifications of the axonal caliber, which could explain a shortening of the axonal life leading to a subsequent secondary degeneration. The authors also described the presence of terminal axonal ovoids in the hypocellular center of chronic active lesions. This cannot be explained by a direct inflammatory insult, but can be related to a continuous "degenerative" process that could be the substrate of the continuous progression characterizing the intermediate and advanced phases of the disease. The clinical observation that in the progressive phase of the disease the spatial distribution of sensory-motor deficits has the classical distal-proximal gradient strongly supports the important role of secondary degenerative processes. This process becomes clinically evident only when the safety factor (number of functioning axons) is joined. Very recently, Lovas et al. [47] performed a postmortem study of the cervical spinal cord in a group of patients with secondary progressive MS. They found that axonal density was reduced both in the plaque and in the normal appearing white matter (NAWM). At least two-thirds of the axons were lost in inactive, chronic lesions. Moreover, axons were thinner in the plaques than in the NAWM. The authors concluded that their observations support the concept of slow axonal degeneration rather than acute damage as a cause of chronic disability. Similar findings (Trapp, personal communication) are consistent with the atrophy of the cervical spinal cord demonstrated in these patients by MRI [48, 49]. The degeneration of axons may depend on the loss of extrinsic trophic factors provided by myelin-forming cells, as has been demonstrated in chronic demyelinative and dysmyelinative disorders. For instance, mutations of the PLP gene cause Pelizaeus Merzbacher disease and spastic paraplegia, characterized by secondary axonal degeneration.

Magnetic Resonance

Some new MR techniques characterized by a better pathological specificity have focused attention on axonal damage in MS. MR spectroscopy [50-54], magnetization transfer imaging [55-58], brain and spinal cord atrophy measures [48, 49, 59, 60], and T1 black holes [61] provided indirect evidence of axonal loss as an early phenomenon in MS. There is a correlation between axonal loss and magnetic transfer ratio (MTR) both in plaques [62] and in NAWM [63]. Diffusion-weighted imaging, MR spectroscopy, and magnetization transfer clearly demonstrated that the normal-appearing white matter is also affected in MS, as a result of the axonal degeneration and probably also because of small foci of inflammatory activity, undetected by conventional MRI techniques [52, 64]. Magnetization transfer histograms of the normal-appearing brain tissue in patients with isolated syndromes revealed subtle changes outside visible lesions whose severity was predictive of the future development of CDMS [65]. Ventricular enlargement is also present in these patients and predicts the future development of CDMS [66]. Of great interest is the observation, in a post hoc analysis of two subgroups of patients participating in the IFNβ-1a (Avonex, Biogen) trial in relapsing-remitting MS, that during the 2nd year the brain atrophy progressed significantly less in the treated group then in the placebo group [67]. A group of untreated patients, in the same trial, underwent corpus callosum and third and lateral ventricles width measurements. Corpus callosum atrophy and ventricular dilatation significantly increased during the 2-year follow-up [68]. The increase of ventricular width was associated with an increase of disability and was predicted by the baseline number of gadolinium-enhancing lesions. These two studies suggest that inflammatory activity contributes to brain atrophy and that the reduction of disease activity reduces the progression of brain atrophy; however, the study duration was too short to allow any definite conclusion and the influence of other factors, like steroid treatment, must be considered.

Previous Clinical Trials

The most-striking evidence of the positive effects of an early anti-inflammatory treatment in MS derives from the Optic Neuritis Treatment Trial (ONTT). The trial demonstrated that a single course of 3 days of 1 g of intravenous methylprednisolone reduced by about 50% the risk at 2 years of conversion to CDMS [69]. The beneficial effect was transitory, being lost at 5 years follow-up [70]. There are some indications that the effects of IFNβ-1a (Rebif, Serono) on disease activity may vary with the disease phase. In the PRISMS study (Prevention of Relapses and Disability by Interferon B-1a Subcutaneously in Multiple Sclerosis) in patients with an EDSS score ≤3.5 at entry, the low and the high dose of IFNβ-1a reduced the clinical and MRI activity to the same extent. In patients with an EDSS score >3.5 the proportion of patients free from exacerbation and with inactive scans was significantly reduced in the high dose only [6]. These data suggest that patients in the early phases of the disease could benefit from lower doses of IFNβ-1a. In the same way, the trial testing glatiramer acetate in relapsing-remitting MS [9] showed that the therapeutic effect appeared to be most pronounced in patients with the lowest EDSS score at entry.

The results of two recent double-blind placebo-controlled clinical trials (ETOMS, Early Treatment of Multiple Sclerosis [23] and CHAMPS, Controlled High Risk Subjects Avonex Multiple Sclerosis Prevention Study [71]) are supportive of early treatment of MS.

The European ETOMS trial enrolled 308 patients with onset of first monosymptomatic or polysymptomatic syndromes suggestive of MS no more than 3 months before study entry and with brain MRI suggestive of MS. The patients were randomized to receive 22 µg of IFNβ-1a (Rebif, Serono) by subcutaneous injection once a week or placebo for 2 years. The proportion of patients converting to CDMS was significantly lower for the IFNβ-treated group than for the placebo group (34% vs. 45%, $p=0.047$), with a 24% relative reduction of conversion risk with the active treatment. The time at which 30% of patients had converted to CDMS (occurrence of a second relapse) was 569 days in the IFNβ group and 252 in the placebo group ($p=0.034$). The annual relapse rate was lower in the IFNβ group (0.33) compared with the placebo group (0.43), with a reduction of 23%. There were significantly fewer new T2 lesions in the IFNβ-1a group than in the placebo group ($p<0.001$). The proportion of patients without MRI activity during the study was significantly higher in the IFNβ group than in the placebo group (16% versus 6%, $p=0.005$). At the end of the study, there was an increase in T2 lesion volume of 8.8% in the placebo group compared with the baseline value, while in the IFNβ group there was a decrease of 13% [23].

The American CHAMPS trial enrolled 383 patients with onset of a first monosymptomatic syndrome suggestive of MS no more than 2 weeks before study entry and with a brain MRI suggestive of MS. The patients were randomized to receive 30 µg of IFNβ-1a (Avonex, Biogen), by intramuscular injection once a week or placebo. The proportion of patients converting to CDMS was significantly lower for the IFNβ-treated group than for the placebo group (35% vs. 50%, $p=0.002$). Compared with the patients in the placebo group, patients in the IFNβ-1a group had a relative reduction in the volume of brain lesions on T2-weighted MRI scans ($p<0.001$), fewer new or enlarging lesions on T2-weighted MRI scans ($p<0.001$), and fewer gadolinium-enhancing lesions on T1-weighted scans ($p<0.001$) at 18 months [71].

The effect of IFNβ-1a treatment was slightly greater in CHAMPS than in ETOMS. This difference may be related to differences in the dose administered (30 µg in CHAMPS versus 22 µg in ETOMS) and in the different inclusion criteria. The CHAMPS trial included monosymtpomatic patients, whereas the ETOMS study included both monosymptomatic and polysymptomatic patients, and the risk of conversion was about two times higher for multifocal than unifocal presentation in the ETOMS study. Moreover, the delay between the onset of the first attack and inclusion in the trial was shorter in the CHAMPS study (2 weeks) than in the ETOMS study (3 months), and this difference could lead to subtly different populations. The median T2 lesion volume at baseline was higher in the ETOMS than in the CHAMPS study, suggesting a more severe group in the ETOMS study. The data of these two trials strongly support the idea that early treatment could modify disease course.

Conclusions

The clinical, immunopathological, and imaging data suggest that the early treatment of MS patients with immunomodulatory drugs is advantageous compared with treatment started later in the disease course. Since disability accumulated in the first 5 years after onset corresponds roughly to three-quarters of the disability status after 15 years, the early reduction of relapse rate as well as of the extent of pathological lesions should be the strategy for patients. Early treatment has a robust rationale both in preventing irreversible changes and in reducing clinical and MRI activities with favorable prognostic implications.

All patients with a diagnosis of definite MS who are in an active phase of the disease are candidates for treatment. Patients with relapsing-remitting MS who have already accumulated some degree of disability and who have evidence of disease activity require immediate treatment. Patients with an evident benign course or with long-standing quiescent disease should also be treated if they experience recurrent clinical relapses. The decision is somewhat more difficult in relapsing-remitting MS patients who do not have clinical disability but who present a clinical relapse after a long period of clinical activity. In these cases it is important to perform brain MRI to determine whether the treatment is required. There are strong arguments that suggest using brain MRI in order to decide when treatment should be started. It is at least 10 times more sensitive in revealing disease activity than clinical evaluation, the number of active lesions on MRI is predictive of short- and long-term disease clinical activity, and every new brain lesion can cause permanent brain damage. Moreover, the new diagnostic criteria recently published [72], based on the repeat of MRI 3 and 6 months after the first attack suggestive of MS, will allow us to anticipate the diagnosis of definite MS in most patients.

There are still some concerns about the long-term advantages of the early treatment of MS. Detractors of this strategy claim that there are no proofs that long term disability is influenced by the positive effects of immunomodulatory treatment on disease activity. The 4-year data of the ETOMS study, available soon, will help to clarify these doubts.

References

1. Confavreux C, Aimard G, Devic M (1980) Course and prognosis of multiple sclerosis assessed by the computerized data processing of 349 patients. Brain 103:281-300
2. Weinshenker BG, Bass B, Rice GPA, Noseworthy J, Carriere W, Baskerville J, Ebers GC (1989) The natural history of multiple sclerosis: a geographically based study. Clinical course and disability. Brain 112:133-146

3. The IFNB MS Study Group (A) (1993) Interferon Beta-1b is effective in relapsing-remitting multiple sclerosis. I. Clinical results of a multicenter, randomized, double-blind, placebo-controlled trial. Neurology 43:655-661

4. Jacobs LD, Cookfair DL, Rudick RA et al (1996) Intramuscular interferon beta-1a for disease progression in relapsing multiple sclerosis. Ann Neurol 39:285-294

5. Rudick RA, Goodkin D, Jacobs L et al (1997) Impact of interferon beta-1a on neurologic disability in relapsing multiple sclerosis. Neurology 49:358-363

6. PRISMS (Prevention of Relapses and Disability by Interferon B-1a Subcutaneously in Multiple Sclerosis) Study Group (1998) Randomised double-blind placebo-controlled study of interferon β-1a in relapsing/remitting multiple sclerosis. Lancet 352:1498-1504

7. The OWIMS Study. The Once Weekly Interferon for MS study Group (OWIMS) (1999) Evidence of interferon β-1a dose response in relapsing-remitting MS. Neurology 53:679-686

8. Johnson KP, Brooks RB, Cohen JA, The Copolymer 1 Multiple Sclerosis Research Group (1995) Copolymer 1 reduces relapse rate and improves disability in relapsing-remitting multiple sclerosis: results of the phase III multicenter, double-blind, placebo-controlled trial. Neurology 45:1268-1276

9. Johnson KP, Brooks RB, Cohen JA, The Copolymer 1 Multiple Sclerosis Research Group (1998) Extended use of glatiramer acetate (Copaxone) is well tolerated and maintains its clinical effect on multiple sclerosis relapse rate and degree of disability. Neurology 50:701-708

10. Comi G, Filippi M, Copaxone MRI Study Group (1999) The effect of glatiramer acetate (Copaxone) on disease activity as measured by cerebral MRI in patients with relapsing-remitting multiple sclerosis (RRMS) Neurology 52:A289

11. European Study Group on Interferon β-1b in Secondary Progressive MS (1998) Placebo multicentre randomised trial of interferon β-1b in treatment of secondary progressive multiple sclerosis. Lancet 352:1491-1497

12. Paty DW on behalf of the SPECTRIMS Study Group (1999) Results of the 3-year, double blind, placebo controlled study of interferon beta- 1a (Rebif) in secondary progressive MS. J Neurol 246 [suppl 1]:I15

13. Report of the Quality Standards Subcommittee of the American Academy of Neurology (1994) Practice advisory on selection of patients with multiple sclerosis for treatment with Betaseron. Neurology 44:1537-1540

14. Lublin FD, Whitaker JN, Eidelman BH, Miller AE, Arnason BGW, Burks JS (1996) Management of patients receiving interferon beta-1b for multiple sclerosis. Neurology 46:12-18

15. Oger J, Freedman M (1999) Consensus Statement of the Canadian MS Clinical Network on: The Use of Disease Modyfing Agents in Multiple Sclerosis. Can J Neurol Sci 26:274-275

16. Polman CH, Miller DH, Mcdonald WI, Thompson AJ (1999) Treatment recommendations for interferon β in multiple sclerosis. J Neurol Neurosurg Psychiatry 67:561-566

17. Rieckman P, Toyka KV, and the Austrian-German-Swiss Multiple Sclerosis Therapy Consensus Group (MSTCG) (1999) Escalating immunotherapy of multiple sclerosis. Eur Neurol 42:121-127

18. Comi G, Martinelli V, Martino G (1998) Early treatment of multiple sclerosis. Eur J Neurol 5 [suppl 2]:S19-S21

19. Rudick AR (1999) Disease-modifying drugs for relapsing remitting multiple sclerosis and future directions for multiple sclerosis therapeutics. Arch Neurol 56:1079-1084

20. Filippi M, Horsfield MA, Morissey SP, MacManus DG, Rudge P, McDonald WI, Miller DH (1994) Quantitative brain MRI lesion load predicts the course of clinically isolated syndromes suggestive of multiple sclerosis. Neurology 44:635-641

21. O'Riordan JI, Thompson AJ, Kingsley PE, MacManus DG, Kendall BE, Rudge P, McDonald WI, Miller DH (1998) The prognostic value of brain MRI in clinically isolated syndromes of the CNS. A 10-year follow-up. Brain 121:495-503

22. Brex PA, O'Riordan JI, Miszkiel KA, Moseley IF, Thompson AJ, Plant GT, Miller DH (1999) Multisequence MRI in clinically isolated syndromes and the early development of MS. Neurology 53:1184-1190

23. Comi G, Filippi M, Barkhof F and the ETOMS Study Group (2001) Effects of early interferon treatment on conversion to definite multiple sclerosis: a randomised study. Lancet 357:1576-1582

24. Lucchinetti C et al (2000) Heterogeneity of multiple sclerosis lesions: implications for the pathogenesis of demyelination. Ann Neurol 47:707-717

25. Soldestrom M, Jin Ya-Ping, Hillert J, Link H (1998) Optic neuritis: prognosis for multiple sclerosis from MRI, CSF, and HLA findings. Neurology 50:708-714

26. Sciacca FL, Ferri C, Vandenbroeck K, Veglia F, Gobbi C, Martinelli F, Franciotta D, Zaffaroni M, Marrosu M, Martino G, Martinelli V, Comi G, Canal N, Grimaldi LMG (1999) Relevance of interleukin 1 receptor antagonist intron 2 polymorphism in Italian MS. Neurology 52:1896-1898

27. Weinshenker BG (1994) Natural history of multiple sclerosis. Ann Neurol 36 [Suppl]: S6-S11

28. Runmarker B, Andersen O (1993) Prognostic factors in a multiple sclerosis incidence cohort with twenty-five years of follow-up. Brain 116:117-134

29. Yu BM, Johnson MJ, Tuohy VK (1996) A predictable sequential determinant spreading cascade invariably accompanies progression of experimental autoimmune encephalomyelitis: a basis for peptide-specific therapy after onset of clinical disease. J Exp Med 183:1777-1788

30. Thuoy VK, Weinstock-Guttman B, Kinkel RP (1997) Diversity and plasticity of self recognition during the development of multiple sclerosis. J Clin Invest 99:1682-1690

31. Balashov KE, Smith DR, Khoury SJ, Hafler DA, Weiner HL (1997) Increased interleukin 12 production in progressive multiple sclerosis: induction by activated CD4+ T cells via CD40 ligand. Proc Natl Acad Sci U S A 94:599-603

32. Nicoletti F et al (1996) Elevated serum levels of interleukin-12 in chronic progressive multiple sclerosis. Neuroimmunology 70:87-90

33. Lucchinetti CF, Bruck W, Rodriguez M, Lassmann H (1996) Distinct patterns of multiple sclerosis pathology indicates heterogeneity on pathogenesis. Brain Pathol 6:259-274

34. Lassmann H (1998) Neuropathology in multiple sclerosis: new concepts. Mult Scler 4:93-98

35. Bo L et al (1994) Induction of nitricoxide synthase in demyeinating regions of multiple sclerosis brains. Ann Neurol 36:778-786

36. Charcot JM (1868) Histologie de la sclerose en plaques. Gaz Hop (Paris) 141:554-558

37. Putnam TJ (1936) Studies in multiple sclerosis. Arch Neurol Psychol 35:1289-1308

38. Greenfield J, King L (1936) Observations on the histopathology of the cerebral lesions in disseminated sclerosis. Brain 59:445-458

39. Prineas WJ, Barnard RO, Revesz T, Kwon EE, Sharer L, Cho ES (1993) Multiple sclerosis. Pathology of recurrent lesions. Brain 116:681-693

40. Rodriguez et al (1992) Central nervous system demyelination and remyelination in multiple sclerosis and viral models of disease. J Neuroimmunol 40:255-263

41. Bruck W, Schmied M, Suchanek G, Bruck Y, Breitschopf H, Poser S et al (1994) Oligodendrocytes in the early course of multiple sclerosis. Ann Neurol 35:65-73

42. Ozawa K, Suchanek G, Breitschopf H, Bruck W, Budka H, Jellinger K, Lassmann H (1994) Patterns of oligodendroglia pathology in multiple sclerosis. Brain 117:1311-1322

43. Linington C, Engelhardt B, Kapocs G, Lassmann H (1992) Induction of persistenly demyelinated lesions in the rat following the repeated adoptive transfer of encephalitogenic T cells and demyelinating antibody. J Neuroimmunol 40:219-224

44. Ferguson B, Matyszak MK, Esiri MM, Perry VH (1997) Axonal damage in acute multiple sclerosis lesions. Brain 120:393-399
45. Trapp BD, Peterson J, Ransohoff RM, Rudick R, Mork S, Bo L (1998) Axonal transection in the lesions of multiple sclerosis. New Engl J Med 338:278-285
46. Raine C, Cannella B, Hauser S, Genain C (1999) Demyelination in primate autoimmune encephalomyelitis and acute multiple sclerosis lesions: a case for antigen-specific antibody mediation. Ann Neurol 46:144-160
47. Lovas G, Szilagyi N, Majtenyi K, Palkovits M, Komoly S (2000) Axonal changes in chronic demyelinated cervical spinal cord plaques. Brain 123:308-317
48. Filippi M, Campi A, Colombo B, Pereira C, Martinelli V, Baratti C, Comi G (1996) A spinal cord MRI study of benign and secondary progressive multiple sclerosis. J Neurol 243(7):502-505
49. Losseff NA, Webb SL, O'Riordan JI, Page R, Wang L, Barker GJ, Tofts PS, McDonald WI, Miller DH, Thompson AJ (1996) Spinal cord atrophy and disability in multiple sclerosis. A new reproducible and sensitive MRI method with potential to monitor disease progression. Brain 119:701-708
50. Narayana PA, Doyle TJ, Lai D, Wolinsky JSM (1998) Serial proton magnetic resonance spectroscopic imaging, contrast-enhanced magnetic resonance imaging, and quantitative lesion volumetry in multiple sclerosis. Ann Neurol 43:56-71
51. Tourbah A, Stievenart JL, Gout O, Fontaine B, Liblau R, Lubetzki C, Cabanis EA, Lyon-Caen O (1999) Localized proton magnetic resonance spectroscopy in relapsing remitting versus secondary progressive multiple sclerosis. Neurology 53:1091-1097
52. Sarchielli P, Presciutti O, Pelliccioli GP, Tarducci R, Gobbi G, Chiarini P, Alberti A, Vicinanza F, Gallai V (1999) Absolute quantification of brain metabolites by proton magnetic resonance spectroscopy in normal-appearing white matter of multiple sclerosis patients. Brain 122:513-521
53. Matthews PM, De Stefano N, Narayanan S, Francis GS, Wolinsky JS, Antel JP, Arnold DL (1998) Putting magnetic resonance spectroscopy studies in context: axonal damage and disability in multiple sclerosis. Semin Neurol 18:327-336
54. Falini A, Calabrese G, Filippi M, Origgi D, Lipari S, Colombo B, Comi G, Scotti G (1998) Benign versus secondary-progressive multiple sclerosis: the potential role of proton MR spectroscopy in defining the nature of disability. Am J Neuroradiol 19:223-229
55. Rocca MA, Mastronardo G, Rodegher M, Comi G, Filippi M (1999) Long-term changes of magnetization transfer-derived measures from patients with relapsing-remitting and secondary progressive multiple sclerosis. Am J Neuroradiol 20:821-827
56. Davie CA, Silver NC, Barker GJ, Tofts PS, Thompson AJ, McDonald WI, Miller DH (1999) Does the extent of axonal loss and demyelination from chronic lesions in multiple sclerosis correlate with the clinical subgroup? J Neurol Neurosurg Psychiatry 67:710-715
57. Filippi M, Rocca MA, Minicucci L, Martinelli V, Ghezzi A, Bergamaschi R, Comi G (1999) Magnetization transfer imaging of patients with definite MS and negative conventional MRI. Neurology 52:845-848
58. Brochet B, Dousset V (1999) Pathological correlates of magnetization transfer imaging abnormalities in animal models and humans with multiple sclerosis. Neurology 53 [Suppl 3]:S127
59. Rudick RA, Fisher E, Lee JC, Simon J, Jacobs L (1999) Use of the brain parenchymal fraction to measure whole brain atrophy in relapsing-remitting MS. Multiple Sclerosis Collaborative Research Group. Neurology 53:1698-1704
60. Dastidar P, Heinonen T, Lehtimaki T, Ukkonen M, Peltola J, Erila T, Laasonen E, Elovaara I (1999) Volumes of brain atrophy and plaques correlated with neurological disability in secondary progressive multiple sclerosis. J Neurol Sci 165:36-42

61. van Waesberghe JH, Kampphorst W, De Groot CJ, van Walderveen MA, Castelijns JA, Ravid R, Lycklama à Nijeholt G, van der Valk P, Polman C, Thompson AJ, Barkhof F (1999) Axonal loss in multiple sclerosis lesions: magnetic resonance imaging insights into substrates of disability. Ann Neurol 46:747-754

62. Gass A et al (1994) Correlation of magnetization transfer ratio with disability in multiple sclerosis. Ann Neurol 36:62-67

63. Filippi M et al (1999) Comparison of MS clinical phenotypes using conventional and magnetization transfer MRI. Neurology 52:588-594

64. Filippi M et al (1995) A magnetization transfer imaging study of normal appearing white matter in multiple sclerosis. Neurology 45:478-482

65. Iannucci G, Tortorella C, Rovaris M, Sormani MP, Comi G, Filippi M (2000) Prognostic value of MR and magnetization transfer imaging findings in patients with clinically isolated syndromes suggestive of multiple sclerosis at presentation. Am J Neuroradiol 21:1034-1038

66. Brex PA et al (2000) Detection of ventricular enlargement in patients at the earliest clinical stage of MS. Neurology 54:1689-1691

67. Rudick RA et al (1999) Use of the brain parenchimal fraction to measure whole brain atrophy in relapsing-remitting MS. Neurology 10:1698-1704

68. Simon JH, Jacobs LD, Campion MK, Rudick RA, Cookfair DL, Herndon RM, Richert JR, Salazar AM, Fisher JS, Goodkin DE, Simonian N, Lajaunie M, Miller DE, Wende K, Martens-Davidson A, Kinkel RP, Munschauer III FE, Brownscheidle and The Multiple Sclerosis Collaborative Research (1999) A longitudinal study of brain atrophy in relapsing multiple sclerosis. Neurology 53:139-148

69. Beck RW, Cleary PA, Trobe JD et al (1993) The effect of corticosteroids for acute optic neuritis on the subsequent development of multiple sclerosis. N Engl J Med 329:1764-1769

70. Optic Neuritis Study Group (1997) The 5-year risk of MS after optic neuritis. Experience of the optic neuritis treatment trial. Neurology 49:1404-1413

71. Jacobs LD, Beck RW, Simon JH and the CHAMPS Study Group (2000) Intramuscular interferon b-1a therapy initiated during a first demyelinating event in multiple sclerosis. N Engl J Med 343:898-904

72. McDonald WI, Compston A, Edan G et al (2001) Recommended diagnostic criteria for multiple sclerosis: guidelines from the international panel on the diagnosis of multiple sclerosis. Ann Neurol 50:121-127

Inflammation, Demyelination, and Axonal Degeneration: Three Aspects of the Pathogenesis of Multiple Sclerosis Revealed by Campath-1H Treatment

A.J. COLES, M.G. WING, P. MOLYNEUX, A. PAOLILLO, C.M. DAVIE, G. HALE, D. MILLER, H. WALDMANN, A. COMPSTON

Introduction

It is hard to account for all the features of multiple sclerosis by episodes of demyelination and remyelination alone: the rapidity of recovery from a relapse, for instance, or the transition from relapsing-remitting disease to progressive accumulation of disability. Here, we report observation from the close study of a small number of patients treated with an experimental agent, Campath-1H, that cast some light on these issues.

Campath-1H is a humanized monoclonal antibody that targets the CD52 antigen and causes a prolonged T lymphopenia after one pulse. The rationale for its use in based on the finding that similar antibody treatment in mice causes long-term allograft acceptance [1, 2]. Our aim was to mimic this laboratory effect by administering Campath-1H to patients with active multiple sclerosis and induce long-lasting tolerance to the antigen(s) driving their inflammation. A pilot study of 7 patients had shown that Campath-1H reduces magnetic resonance imaging (MRI) markers of cerebral inflammation for at least 6 months [3]. We sought in the current study to establish its effect on clinical markers of disease activity.

A surprising observation of our pilot study was that the initial dose of Campath-1H caused a transient and often severe, but invariably reversible, reactivation of previous neurologial relapses that lasted for a few hours. We subsequently established that Campath-1H induced a coincident rise in serum tumor necrosis factor (TNF)-α and interferon (IFN)-γ [4]. Since TNF-α mediates the systemic first-dose effect of OKT3, an anti-CD3 monoclonal antibody [5], we investigated the contribution of TNF-α to the first-dose effect of Campath-1H by in vivo TNF-α neutralization. These results have been reported elsewhere in part [6].

Materials and Methods

Patients and Treatment

Patients were initially selected for treatment if they had clinically definite secondary progressive multiple sclerosis, historical evidence for a sustained deterioration in disability of a least one point in the Kurtzke expandend disability status scale (EDSS) [7] over the preceding year, and at least one new enhancing lesion on a series of 4-monthly gadolinium-enhanced magnetic resonance scans. Of 130 patients screened, 50 fulfilled these clinical criteria, of whom 37 entered screening and 33 met the MRI entry criterion. Of these, 4 patients opted to be open controls for the study and underwent the same follow-up and imaging schedule. Of the 29 treated patients, 1 was treated but later lost to follow-up and has therefore been excluded from the analysis. The remaining 28 patients were reviewed every 3 months and assessed by the same investigator on each occasion (A.J.C.); their mean age was 38.4 years, mean disease duration 12.5 years, and mean EDSS at entry was 5.4. The trial protocol was approved by the Local Research Ethics Committee (LREC 92/49). Radiological markers of tissue destruction were available in 27 patients.

All 29 patients received Campath-1H. On the grounds that an additional CD4 blockade might promote tolerance induction, 14 patients were also randomized subsequently to receive a humanized non-depleting anti-CD4 antibody (Therapeutic Antibody Centre, Oxford). These two treatment groups were further divided into three arms, based on pre-treatment of the first dose of Campath-1H, one cohort received nothing; the second was pre-treated with methylprednisolone and the third was given a soluble TNF-α receptor (a fusion protein of the two TNF-α receptor domains and a human IgG1 constant region, Therapeutic Antibody Centre, Oxford) before the initial dose of Campath-1H. There were therefore six different treatment schedules too which patients were randomized, with 5 patients in each group (except the cohort receiving soluble TNF-α receptor and anti-CD4, in which there were only 4). Each patient was given a total of 100 mg Campath-1H over 5 consecutive days, as a daily 20-mg infusion lasting 4 h. A total of 200 mg of anti-CD4 antibody was given over the subsequent 5 days in 14 patients. Pre-treatment in each group was either with methylprednisolone (500 mg), soluble TNF-α receptor (4 mg), or nothing, given 30 min before the first dose of Campath-1H.

TNF-α assays

Two ELISAs were used to discriminate between free and bound TNF-α. A commercial ELISIA (R&D) detected both free and bound TNF-α, whereas free TNF-α only was detected as follows (data not shown). MicroELISA plates (Dynatech M129B, 96 wells) were coated with anti-human TNF-α antibody (prepared from the 2-179-E11 hybridomas, 1 mg/ml in carbonate-bicarbonate buffer, pH 9.6) and the TNF-α captured from sera samples was reacted with polyclonal goat anti-TNF-α (R&D, 1/500), then anti-goat IgG antibody conjugated with alkaline phosphatase (Sigma, 2 mg/ml) and p-nitrophenol phosphate (Sigma, 1 mg/ml in diethanolamine buffer, pH 9.8), and the optical density read at 405 nm in an automated reader (Bio-Rad 3550). Standard curves were constructed using logit-log transformations and levels of sensitivity determined as the lowest cytokine concentration at which the 95% confidence levels lay above the background optical density, which was 30-60 pg/ml. Bioactive

TNF-α was measurd by the cytotoxic effect of serum (at 1:20) on the L929 cell line [8, 9]. There was a considerable srum effect that disallowed absolute estimations of bioactive TNF-α concentrations; the results are shown as the counts per minute of incorporated ^{3}H for sera taken at different times after Campath-1H, expressed as a percentage of the counts per minute induced by the pre-treatment serum sample. Thus, a fall in the percentage represents an increase in bioactive TNF-α.

Magnetic Resonance Imaging

Scans were performed on a 1.5 system (Signa, GE Medical Systems, Milwaukee, USA) according to a standard protocol [3]. Patients had four scans monthly prior to treatment, then a further six scans monthly immediately after treatment. No imaging was performed between months 6 and 12 after Campath-1H; then patients had seven scans from months 12 to 18. The number of gadolinium DTPA-enhancing lesions demonstrated on the first scan was recorded and the definition of disease activity confined to new enhancing lesions appearing on subsequent investigations. Persistent enhancement in areas that had been active on the previous scan was not counted as a new lesion. For statistical analysis, the study period was divided into five blocks of three informative scans (pre-treatment and months 1-3, 4-6, 13-15, and 16-18 after treatment) and the total number of new enhancing lesions in these blocks was calculated for each patient. To compare activity in patients before and after treatment, we performed a two-tailed signed rank sum test on the logarithm of the ratio between the treatment and baseline blocks.

Brain volume was also derived from MRI. Having ensured acceptable repositioning between images, four contiguous slices from each scan were compared by an established technique [10] and an estimate of the brain volume derived. Changes in cerebral volume between scans were accepted as significant if they fell outside the 95% confidence limits for measurement variation. Wilcoxon matched pairs signed ranks were used for comparing volumes between groups and the Friedman test was used to compare cerebral volumes at different time points.

MRI spectroscopy was performed in patients from a volume of normal-appearing periventricular parietal white matter, ranging in size from 3.5 to 8 ml. This was compared with a voxel in the same region in an identical number of age-matched controls. Water-suppressed ^{1}H spectra were obtained using a 90°-180°-180° sequence for volume selection and spectroscopic acquisition parameters of TE 30 ms, TR 3,000 ms, with 192 averages collected in 10 min using an eight-step phase cycle. Spectra were anlyzed using the LC Model method, which analyzes the in vivo spectrum as a linear combination of a basis set of complete model spectra of metabolite solutions in the frequency domain in vitro and allows distinction between the *N*-acetyl aspartate and *N*-acetyl aspartyl glutamate components to the *N*-acetyl-derived spectra. Spearman's rank correlation test was used to test the data.

Results

TNF-α Does not Mediate the First-Dose Effect of Campath-1H

The first dose of Campath-1H induced a syndrome of urticaria, pyrexia, and rigors. The neurological exacerbations experienced by patients lasted a few hours, were fully reversible, and consisted either of an exacerbation of existing deficits or the reawakening of previously experienced symptoms that may have been quiescent for several years. The neurological exacerbations induced by Campath-1H were not due to de novo inflammation, as there was no change in gadolinium enhancement on MRI before and during the first dose of Campath-1H in two patients pretreated with soluble TNF-α receptor (data not shown).

We randomized patients to receive an infusion either of methylprednisolone (500 mg), soluble TNF-α receptor (4 mg), or no additional therapy before the first dose of Campath-1H, in order to determine the contribution of TNF-α to the transient neurological deterioration seen with the first dose of Campath-1H. Corticosteroids and soluble TNF-α receptor each abolished the rise in free serum TNF-α induced by Campath-1H, but only corticosteroids abolished the systemic response and the neurological deterioration [6].

Inflammation and Demyelination Cause Relapses

Mechanisms underlying the expression of novel symptomatology in multiple sclerosis appear to differ from those that lead to return of previously experienced symptoms. Defining relapse as the appearance of any symptom or sign, including the exacerbation of pre-existing manifestations, for 24 h or more [11], yielded a total of 9 episodes in the treated group over the 3 months prior to treatment and 15 in the subsequent 18 months. This represents a significant reduction in the annualized relapse rate from 1.24 to 0.34 relapses per patients per year. However, all events experienced by patients beyond the first 2 months after Campath-1H consisted of a transient worsening of pre-existing symptoms or signs, lasting no more that 3 days; no treated patient experienced a new clinical manifestation of multiple sclerosis during the follow-up period (Fig. 1a). As expected, the untreated controls had continued relapses.

The most-sensitive marker of cerebral inflammation in multiple sclerosis is the number of gadolinium-enhancing lesions on MRI. Patients had monthly scans for 3 months before and 6 months after Campath-1H, followed by a further series of monthly scans at months 12-18 after treatment to assess the duration of effect. Compared with the 3-month period before Campath-1H, the number of enhancing magnetic resonance lesions was suppressed throughout the 18-month follow-up period in all the treated patients: by 72% in the first 3 months after treatment, by 90% between months 3 and 6, by 66% over months 12-15, and by 71% in the final 3 months (Fig. 1b, $p<0.001$). None of the treatments for

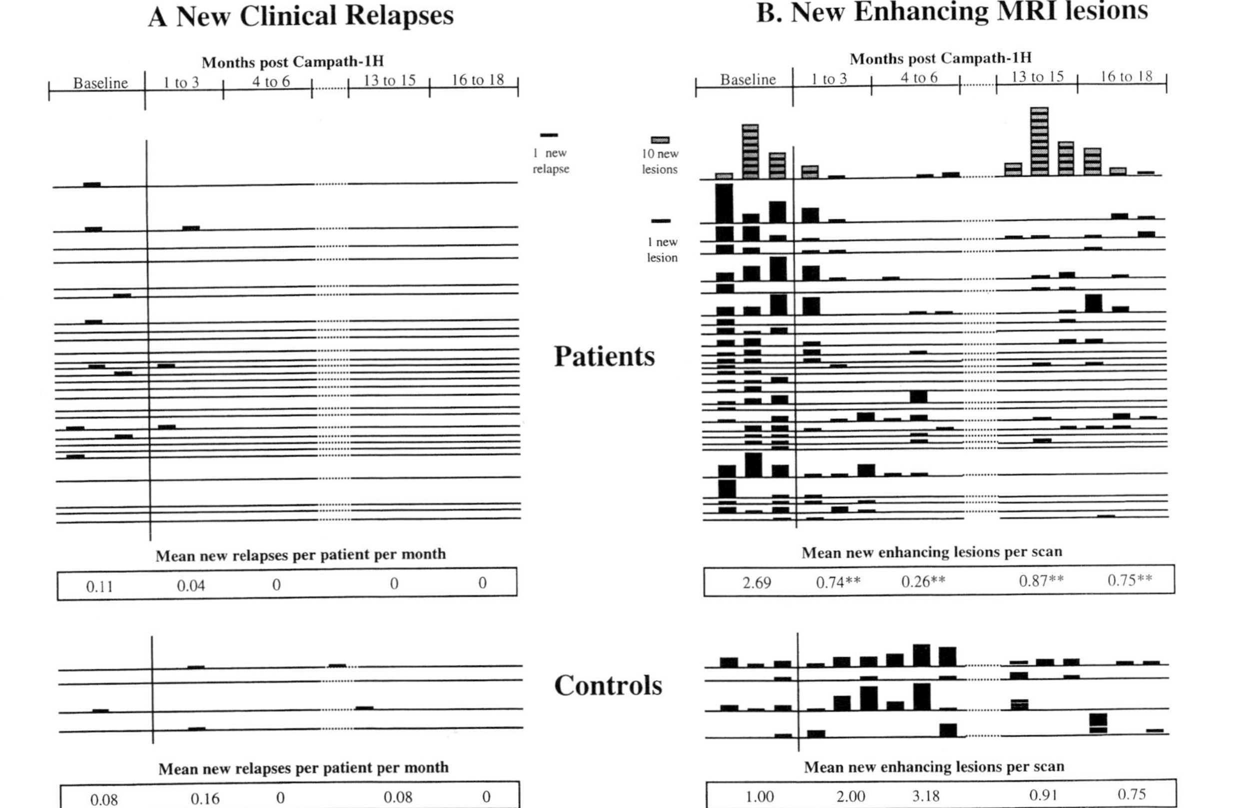

Fig. 1. Disease activity in 28 patients with multiple sclerosis after Campath-1H treatment, shown as **a** new clinical relapses and **b** the number of new gadolinium-enhancing magnetic resonance imaging lesions in each patient. The *length of the bars* indicates the duration of observation for each individual (★★★ $p<0.001$)

the first-dose effect nor anti-CD4 antibody treatment had any effect on this suppression of new lesions. This trend was observed in every patient, but 1 patient weights the absolute mean value of new enhancing lesions per scan with ten times more active disease before and after treatment.

Clinical Progression and Axonal Degeneration

Defining progression of disability as an increase in the EDSS of 1 point over 3 months (or 0.5 points when the EDSS is greater than 5.5), 15 of 28 patients deteriorated in the 18 months after treatment (Fig. 2a). Therefore, some patients continued to acquire disability, not by the accumulation of new lesions, but by progression of existing deficit. The 13 patients with progressive disability had a smaller mean brain volume before treatment (Fig. 2b, $p=0.05$) and a significantly higher rate of volume loss compared with those with stable disability (-6.7 ml/year compared with -0.7 ml/year; $p=0.009$). This was shown to be due to axonal degeneration by MRI spectroscopy for N-acetyl aspartate [6]. This group of patients with progresssive disability had a higher MRI inflammatory load before treatment with Campath-1H ($p<0.001$) compared with those with stable disability. Although there was a small, but significant, difference in inflammatory load for the subsequent 18 months between patients with stable or progressive disability, the reduction in inflammation by Campath-1H was equivalent between the two groups of patients (Fig. 2c).

No clinical parameter before treatment discriminated patients who subsequently developed progressive cerebral atrophy; neither did treatment of the first-dose effect, nor the addition of monoclonal anti-CD4 antibody, influence clinical progression or cerebral atrophy after treatment with Campath-1H.

Discussion

The rapidity of recovery, at least in part, from a relapse of multiple sclerosis suggests that part of the deficit may be physiological rather than structural. Indeed, evidence already exists for a direct role of inflammation in symptom production; visual evoked potentials in acute optic neuritis are both reduced in amplitude and increased in latency, indicating conduction block and demyelination, and there is gadolinium enhancement on MRI, implying active inflammation; after enhancement ceases, the amplitude of visual evoked potentials returns to normal, suggesting restoration of conduction but the latency of the visual evoked potential remains delayed, implying persistent demyelination [12]. The first-dose effect of Campath-1H, in which we observed a transient reversal of previous or current symptoms due to conduction block coincident with a rise in serum cytokines [4], allows for the mechanisms underlying this effect to be probed. We have excluded free TNF-α as the mediator of the first-dose effect; recent experimental studies implicate nitric oxide as a potential

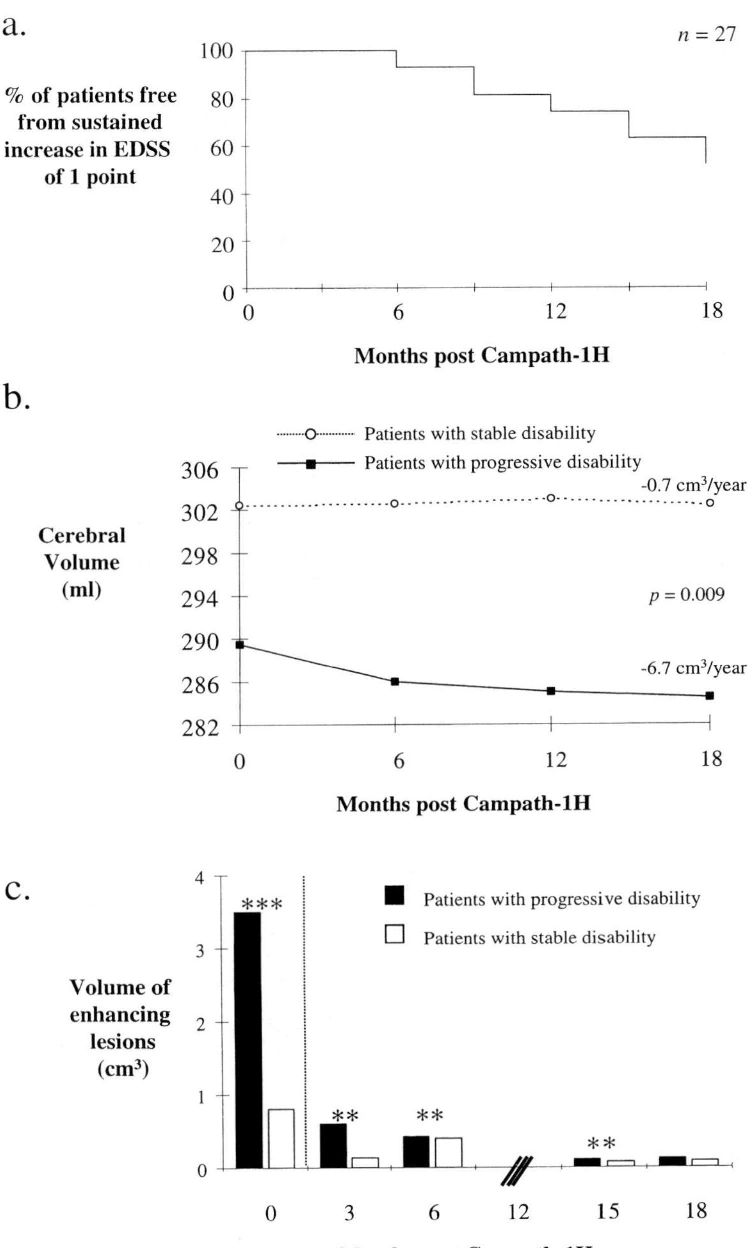

Fig. 2. a The probability of remaining free from clinical progression after Campath-1H and b the cerebral volume of patients who remained clinically stable (*dotted line*) and those who had significant progression (*filled line*) after Campath-1H. c The volume o magnetic resonance imaging gadolinium-enhancing lesions in the patients who remained clinically stable (*white bars*) and those who had significant progression (*filled bars*) after treatment (*** $p<0.001$, ** $p<0.01$)

cause [13]. Whatever its identity, it seems reasonable to suggest that it is induced by inflammation, as well as by lymphocyte depletion following Campath-1H. Thus the mechanism of acute relapse in multiple sclerosis may include fully reversible physiological conduction block caused by mediators of inflammation as well as demyelination.

The radiological data suggest that new gadolinium-enhancing MRI lesion formation is profoundly reduced by a single 5-day pulse of Campath-1H at 3-6 months after treatment and remains significantly suppressed for at least 18 months, to similar levels as seen in patients treated continuously with IFN-β [14-16]. Although this study was only poorly controlled, comparison with a natural history study of the rate of new lesion formation in untreated patients with secondary progressive multiple sclerosis [17] leaves little doubt that the extent of suppression of new enhancing lesions after Campath-1H is a real treatment effect and not simply regression to mean. Gadolinium enhancement in MRI of the brain has been shown experimentally [18], in one human post-mortem study [19] and in a recent pathological study [20], to be associated with inflammation. Taken with the clinical evidence that new neurological sites are not involved after treatment, this supports the current consensus that inflammation, and thereby demyelination, are the pathological mechanisms underlying neurological relapses in multiple sclerosis.

Despite the substantial reduction of MRI disease activity and abolition of new clinical relapses, half of our patients continued to experience deterioration is disability after Campath-1H. Those who deteriorated clinically after Campath-1H had a significantly greater pre-treatment inflammatory load, measured by MRI; they had smaller cerebral volume, and clinical progression correlated significantly with additional cerebral atrophy. Similar progressive cerebral atrophy has been noted in some [21], but not all [22], studies of relapsing-remitting patients treated with IFN-β. This suggests dissociation between the mechanisms underlying cerebral atrophy and gadolinium enhancement. Our work, reported elsewhere [6], suggests that this cerebral atrophy is due to axonal degeneration.

From a therapeutic perspective, it is critical to know whether inflammation precedes, and conditions, subsequent axonal degeneration or if the two processes arise at the same time and proceed independently. In other words, is multiple sclerosis an inflammatory disease with secondary neurodegeneration or is it a primary degenerative disease with additional inflammation? Our study supports the former view, since patients with a high inflammatory load were more likely to subsequently experience axonal degeneration.

Several potential mechanisms can be offered for the progression of axonal degeneration in the absence of active inflammation. It may be a delayed expression of axonal damage sustained during the acute inflammatory phase [23, 24]. Alternatively it may be a consequence of immune deviation towards the Th2 phenotype induced by Campath-1H, as evidenced by downregulation of the expression of IFN-γ by peripheral blood mononuclear cells for at least 12 months, a progressive increase in B cell numbers, and autoimmune hyperthyroidism in one-third of patients treated for multiple sclerosis [25]. As part of this apparent promotion of antibody mediated autoimmunity, anti-neuronal antibodies may have developed, but we found none (data not shown). Lastly, axonal degeneration may be a consequence of demyelination, either through loss of trophic support from the oligodendrocyte [26-28] or secondary to altered electrical conduction [29].

We conclude that inflammation may cause symptoms of multiple sclerosis through demyelination, but also by directly blocking conduction. Clinical progression and brain atrophy are due to axon degeneration; this may continue in the absence of active inflammation, but is conditioned by the amount of prior disease activity. The implication of this analysis, derived from clinical and radiological observations of our patients treated using Campath-1H, supported by observations gathered from a range of pathological and experimental studies, is that anti-inflammatory therapies will best prevent the progression of disability if given early in the course of multiple sclerosis and before the cascade of events that leads to axon degeneration has been irretrievably established.

Acknowledgements. A.J.C. was an MRC Training Fellow and some aspects of this work were supported by a grant from MuSTER. Campath-1H is a registered trademark of Milennium.

References

1. Benjamin RJ, Waldmann H (1986) Induction of tolerance by monoclonal antibody therapy. Nature 320:449-451
2. Qin S, Cobbold SP, Pope H, Helliott J, Kioussis D, Davies J et al (1993) 'Infectious' transplantation tolerance. Science 259:974-977
3. Moreau T, Thorpe J, Miller D, Moseley I, Hale G, Waldmann H et al (1994) Preliminary evidence from magnetic resonance imaging for reduction in disease activity after lymphocyte depletion in multiple sclerosis [published erratum apears in Lancet (1994) 486]. Lancet 344:298-301
4. Moreau T, Coles A, Wing M, Isaacs J, Hale G, Waldmann H et al (1996) Transient increase in symptoms associated with cytokine release in patients with multiple sclerosis. Brain 119:225-237
5. Charpentier B, Hiesse C, Lantz O, Ferran C, Stephens S, O'Shaugnessy D et al (1992) Evidence that antihuman tumor necrosis factor monoclonal antibody prevents OKT3-induced acute syndrome. Transplantation 54:997-1002
6. Coles AJ, Wing M, Molyneux P, Paolillo A, Davies C, Hale G, Miller d, Waldmann H, Compston A (1999) Monoclonal antibody treatment exposes three mechanisms underlying the clinical course of multiple sclerosis. Ann Neurol 46:296-304
7. Kurtzke JF (1983) Rating neurologic impairment in multiple sclerosis: an expanded disability status scale (EDSS). Neurology 33:1444-1452
8. Branch DR, Shah A, Guilbert LJ (1991) A specific and reliable bioassay for the detection of femtomolar levels of human and murine tumor necrosis factors. J Immunol Methods 143:251-261
9. Hay H, Cohen J (1989) Studies on the specificity of the L929 cell bioassay for the measurement of tumour necrosis factor. J Clin Lab Immunol 29:151-155

10. Losseff NA, Wang L, Lai HM, Yoo DS, Gawne Cain ML, McDonald WI et al (1996) Progressive cerebral atrophy in multiple sclerosis. A serial MRI study. Brain 119:2009-2019

11. Poser CM, Paty DW, Scheinberg L, McDonald WI, Davis FA, Ebers GC et al (1983) New diagnostic criteria for multiple sclerosis: guidelines for research protocols. Ann Neurol 13:227-231

12. Youl BD, Turano G, Miller DH, Towell AD, MacManus DG, Moore SG et al (1991) The pathophysiology of acute optic neuritis. An association of gadolinium leakage with clinical and electrophysiological deficits. Brain 114:2437-2450

13. Redford EJ, Kapoor R, Smith KJ (1997) Nitric oxide donors reversibly block axonal conduction:demyelinated axons are especially susceptible. Brain 120:2149-2157

14. Stone LA, Frank JA, Albert PS, Bash CN, Calabresi PA, Maloni H et al (1997) Characterization of MRI response to treatment with interferon beta-1b: contrast-enhancing MRI lesion frequency as a primary outcome measure. Neurology 49:862-869

15. Rudge P, Miller D, Crimlisk H, Thorpe J (1995) Does interferon beta cause initial exacerbation of multiple sclerosis? (letter) Lancet 345:580

16. Stone LA, Albert PS, Smith ME, De Carli C, Armstrong MR, McFarlin DE et al (1995) Changes in the amount of diseased white matter over time in patients with relapsing-remitting multiple sclerosis. Neurology 45:1808-1814

17. Molyneux PD, Filippi M, Barkhof F, Gasperini C, Yousry TA, Truyen L et al (1998) Correlations between monthly enhanced MRI lesion rate and changes in T2 lesion volume in multiple sclerosis. Ann Neurol 43:332-339

18. Hawkins CP, Mackenzie F, Tofts P, du Boulay EP, McDonald WI (1991) Patterns of blood-brain barrier breakdown in inflammatory demyelination. Brain 114:801-810

19. Katz D, Taubenberger JK, Cannella B, McFarlin DE, Raine CS, McFarland HF (1993) Correlation between magnetic resonance imaging findings and lesion development in chronic, active multiple sclerosis. Ann Neurol 34:661-669

20. Bruck W, Bitsch A, Kolenda H, Bruck Y, Stiefel M, Lassmann H (1997) Inflammatory central nervous system demyelination: correlation of magnetic resonance imaging findings with lesion pathology. Ann Neurol 42:783-793

21. Molyneux PD, Kappos L, Polman C, Pozzilli C, Barkhof F, Filippi M, Yousry T, Hahn D, Wagner K, Ghazi M, Beckmann K, Dahlke F, Losseff N, Barker GJ, Thompson AJ, Miller DH (2000) The effect of interferon beta-1b treatment on MRI measures of cerebral atrophy in secondary progressive multiple sclerosis. European Study Group on interferon beta-1b in secondary progressive multiple sclerosis. Brain 123:2256-2263

22. Rudick RA, Fisher E, Lee JC, Simon J, Jacobs L (1999) Use of the brain parenchymal fraction to measure whole brain atrophy in relapsing-remitting MS. Multiple Sclerosis Collaborative Research Group. Neurology 53:1698-1704

23. Ferguson B, Matyszak MK, Perry VH (1997) Axonal damage in acute multiple sclerosis lesions. Brain 120:393-399

24. Trapp BD, Peterson J, Ransohoff RM, Rudick RA, Mork S, Bo L (1998) Axonal transection in the lesions of multiple sclerosis. N Engl J Med 338:278-285

25. Coles A, Wing M, Smith S, Corradu F, Greer S, Taylor C, Weetman A, Hale G, Chatterjee VK, Waldmann H, Compston A (1999) Pulsed monoclonal antibody treatment modulates T cell responses in multiple sclerosis but induces autoimmune thyroid disease. Lancet 354:1691-1695

26. Colello RJ, Pott U, Schwab ME (1994) The role of oligodendrocytes and myelin on axon maturation in the developing rat retinofugal pathway. J Neurosci 14:2594-2605

27. Kaplan MR, Meyer Franke A, Lambert S, Bennett V, Duncan ID, Levinson SR et al (1997) Induction of sodium channel clustering by oligodendrocytes. Nature 386:724-728

28. Meyer Franke A, Kaplan MR, Pfrieger FW, Barres BA (1995) Characterization of the signaling interactions that promote the survival and growth of developing retinal ganglion cells in culture. Neuron 15:805-819
29. Pfrieger FW, Barres BA (1997) Synaptic efficacy enhanced by glial cells in vitro. Science 277:1684-1687

Genetic Regulation of Nerve Cell Death/Glial Activation and Protective Effects of Myelin Basic Protein Autoimmune Neurotrophin Production in Mechanically Induced Neurodegeneration

F. Piehl, O. Lidman, T. Olsson

Genetics of Multiple Sclerosis and Experimental Autoimmune Encephalomyelitis

The critical pathogenic steps leading to clinical multiple sclerosis (MS) are generally believed to be regulated by several different genes, with five to ten genes theoretically having a major impact on disease susceptibility [1-3]. This is supported by epidemiological data demonstrating a considerable lowering of concordance rates from monozygotic to dizygotic twins [4]. It has been known for approximately 30 years that certain haplotypes of the HLA gene region predispose for MS. In particular, individuals carrying HLA DR2 (DRB1*1501-DRB5*0101-DQA1*0102-DQB1*0602) are at higher risk. HLA DR3 provides some risk increase, while in certain populations DR4 may be important [5, 6]. So far the HLA complex remains the only well-established genome region known to influence MS [4, 7-9], in spite of the fact that estimations of the relative genetic risk conveyed by the HLA complex alone vary between 5% and 60% [7, 10, 11]. Notably, no single HLA type seems to exclude MS. It is therefore clear that as yet unidentified genes residing outside the HLA must also be of importance for disease susceptibility in MS.

The HLA system can be described as a cluster of many genes regulating immunity. Since the genes within the major histocompatibility complex (MHC) are in strong linkage disequilibrium, i.e., they are inherited *en bloc* with a much lower degree of recombination than in other parts of the genome, it is very difficult to genetically dissect the effect of the HLA on MS. In the rat, whose MHC is termed RT1, MHC regulation of experimental autoimmune encephalomyelitis (EAE) has mostly been described as all-or-none phenomenum, as would be the case if it mainly determined the ability of presentation of a certain peptide autoantigen. However, recent studies employing inbred rat strains in which the entire genome is kept constant with exception for the MHC demonstrate that the MHC seems to regulate the degree of disease susceptibility and different features of the disease phenotype in a more-complex way, for example by regulating the ease with which an environmental factor triggers disease [12]. By using rat strains with MHC recombinations it has been possible to map a major determinant of the MHC influence in particular EAE models to the class II region, which suggests that polymorphisms in B or D molecules (corresponding to the human DQ and DR molecules, respectively) are of importance in regulating the encephalitogenicity of the autoanti-genic immune response. However, the existence of regulatory influences from the class I and III regions also became clear from these studies. It is more diffi-cult to speculate about the exact nature of this influence without further study characterization, but genes with important immunoregulatory roles, such as the pro-inflammatory cytokine tumor necrosis factor-α (TNF-α), non-classical class I molecules, and myelin oligodendrocyte glycoprotein (MOG), are obvi-ous candidates.

Linkage studies in the human suggest that non-HLA genes also regulate disease susceptibility. Current data indicate that many genes are involved, but that each gene contributes to only a small degree, thus making traditional linkage studies in a genetically heterogeneous MS group extremely cumber-some [13]. However, the notion of important regulatory effects of non-HLA/MHC genes is strongly supported by genetic studies in rodents, in which genetic heterogeneity can be reduced and variation in environmental influ-ences minimized. During the last four years several studies describing non-MHC gene effects on various EAE phenotypes in the rat have been published [12, 14-19]. More than 10 different genetic loci influencing EAE phenotypes have currently been described in mice [20-23]. In most cases these genomic regions include hundreds of genes, of which the vast majority have not been cloned or functionally characterized. It is therefore still premature to specu-late about possible candidate genes. Nonetheless, it is noteworthy that some genetic regions co-localize with regions known to regulate other autoimmune diseases, such as diabetes and arthritis, whereas others, at least for now, are selective for neuroinflammation [17, 24, 25]. The existence of loci co-localiz-ing with other autoimmune diseases suggests the involvement of genes that affect common mechanisms in inflammatory regulation, such as expression of particular cytokines or chemokines with important roles in inflammation, e.g. interleukin-2 (IL-2) [26].

Conversely, it is also possible that disease-regulating genes are target specif-ic. For MS/EAE, such central nervous system (CNS)-specific mechanisms could hypothetically involve particular aspects of the reactivity of microglia or astro-cytes, local cytokine or chemokine production, or even neuronal vulnerability. These target-specific susceptibility features may also be an explanation for the poor correlation between magnetic resonance imaging and neurological deficits in MS [27], suggesting inter-individual differences in neuronal vulner-ability in inflammatory conditions. An intriguing aspect of this is that such mechanisms could be involved in all CNS disorders with inflammatory compo-nents, such as neurodegenerative and cerebrovascular diseases. Evidence for the existence of this type of genetic influence on regulation of CNS-specific inflammatory features has been obtained in various experimental settings using different inbred rat strains, and includes the expression of MHC mole-cules on microglia [28], TNF-α expression in astrocytes [29], and adhesion molecule expression on brain endothelia [30-32]. In addition, differences in microglia and macrophage activation and T lymphocyte recruitment between one inbred (LEW) and one outbred (SD) rat strain in a spinal cord contusion model have been described [33].

Genetics of Target Tissue Vulnerability

With this background we wanted to explore whether there are genetically determined differences in local glial reactivity and neuronal degeneration that could have an impact on susceptibility for neuroinflammation. This question is difficult to address in the EAE model, however, since it is impossible to dissociate genetic effects on the activation and recruitment of immune cells from those that specifically act on the inflammatory responsiveness of the target tissue. Instead we have tried to resolve this issue by using a nerve lesion paradigm. Peripheral nerve transections are accompanied by a retrograde reaction that involves morphological and metabolic changes in axotomized nerve cell bodies [34, 35], as well as several features that are shared with autoimmune or infectious conditions, such as activation of surrounding glia and upregulation of MHC antigens [36-38]. In contrast to more severe or disruptive events imposed on the CNS, the blood brain barrier is only partially compromised and there is a very sparse recruitment of bloodborne cells. By employing a particular nerve lesion model consisting of avulsions of lumbar ventral roots, which leads to a loss of a majority of the lesioned motoneurons [39, 40], it is possible to study the neuroinflammatory response in the context of a neurodegenerative process. This aspect is particularly interesting because of the current interest in mechanisms leading to axonal damage and neurodegeneration in MS. It is also important to note that this type of reaction does not rely on the recognition of specific antigens or other mechanisms that require active involvement of bloodborne cells, since experimental depletion of T cells does not influence the response [41].

In an initial experiment we examined the ventral root avulsion (VRA) response in the two inbred rat strains DA and ACI, which have similar MHC haplotypes (RT1.AV1), but which differ considerably in their susceptibility to EAE [12, 14, 42]. Our results demonstrate that VRA in the DA strain results in a stronger microglial activation, cytokine induction, and a greater degree of motoneuron loss compared with ACI [41]. In contrast, there were no discernible differences between two DA strains with different MHC (RT1.H and RT1.AV1), suggesting that these strain differences are due to a non-MHC gene effect. The inheritance pattern for susceptibility to neuronal loss and glial MHC class II expression after VRA was examined in a limited intercross experiment between ACI and DA [41]. Nerve cell survival ratios and MHC class II expression displayed a similar pattern, with the F1×ACI and F1×DA groups mounting an intermediate response compared with the two parental strains. The continuous distribution pattern of neuronal loss and inflammato-

Table 1. The response to ventral root avulsion (VRA) and susceptibility to experimental autoimmune encephalomyelitis (EAE) in different inbred rat strains presented as an arbitrary scale ranging from low degree/less susceptible (+) to high degree/highly susceptible (+++). Strains that are not susceptible at all have the designation (–). Glial activation was determined at 1 week after the nerve injury, before significant nerve cell loss had occurred, while the degree of nerve cell death was determined at 3 weeks after the nerve injury. It is apparent that, apart from a correlation between the intensity of the glial activation preceding the neuronal loss, there is also some degree of correlation between susceptibility for EAE and local inflammatory activation after VRA, with the only exception being the E3 strain. However, the E3 strain notably displayed the lowest degree of upregulation of MHC class II among the examined strains (*MBP* myelin basic protein, *MOG* myelin oligodendrocyte glycoprotein, *n.d.* not determined)

	Spinal cord lesion, ventral root avulsion			EAE susceptibility	
Rat strain	Nerve cell death	Glial activation	MHC class II expression on microglia	MBP	MOG
DA(RT1.AV1)	+++	+++	+++	+++	+++
E3(RT1.U)	+++	++	(+)	–	n.d.
BN(RT1.N)	++	++	++(+)	–	++
LEW(RT1.AV1)	++	++	++	+++	+++
LEW(RT1.N)	++	++	++	–	+++
ACI(RT1.AV1)	+	+	+	+	–
PVG(RT1.AV1)	+	+	+	+	+

ry response within the F1×ACI and F1×DA groups suggests that there is more than one gene conferring susceptibility for both variables after nerve root avulsion.

A comprehensive study comprising six different inbred rat strains [BN(RT1.N), DA(RT1.AV1), E3(RT1.U), LEW(RT1.AV1), LEW(RT1.N) and PVG(RT1.AV1)] confirmed the observation that the VRA response is genetically regulated (Table 1) [43]. Apart from neuronal loss, several different parameters related to inflammatory activation were assessed, including expression of glial acidic fibrillary protein (activation marker for astrocytes), microglia response factor-1 (activation marker for microglia), complement 3 (expressed in various glial subtypes upon inflammatory activation), MHC class II, and the pro-inflammatory cytokines IL-1β, TNF-α, and interferon-γ (IFN-γ). Interestingly, this revealed that each strain demonstrated a strain-specific pattern in the degree of increase of the different parameters. The DA strain consistently ranked very high in the different inflammatory parameters, whereas PVG ranked low. The LEW strains displayed intermediate responses together with BN and E3. However, the latter two strains also displayed additional and strain-specific features. Thus there was an almost-complete lack of injury induced MHC class II expression in the E3 strain and a high expression of IL-1β in the BN strain, which was several times higher than in the other strains. Interestingly, the extent of neuronal loss was also genetically regulated, ranging from 21% to 43%. Again, phenotypic differences between strains seem to be mainly regulated by non-MHC genes, since LEW strains with different MHC haplotypes had a similar degree of inflammation, whereas the PVG and DA strain, which share the same MHC haplotype, presented the largest differences. These results clearly demonstrate that there are considerable phenotypic differences in the inflammatory response to mechanical CNS injury, that these seem to be regulated mainly by non-MHC genes, and that different aspects of the inflammatory response are regulated by independent mechanisms.

In EAE models the LEW strain is susceptible, DA rat is very susceptible, BN is susceptible using some protocols, and ACI, E3 and PVG are more or less resistant (Table 1). It is therefore of interest to note that there is some degree of correlation between susceptibility for EAE and local inflammatory activation after VRA, with the only exception being the E3 strain. However, whereas the E3 strain demonstrates a robust increase in several inflammatory parameters and a high degree of nerve cell loss, almost no surface expression of MHC class II can be detected. A poor capability of antigen presentation in the target tissue may thus be of importance for the resistance to EAE in this particular strain.

Taken together these data strongly encourage further studies of genetically regulated CNS-specific antigen-independent susceptibility factors for neuroinflammatory disease. This can be achieved with the same genetic approach used in polygenic diseases such as EAE, namely linkage analysis in an F2 cohort. Two inbred strains that display phenotypic differences are bred to produce heterozygous F1 animals. The F1 rats are then brother-sister mated to produce a F2 population, where each individual will carry a mix of the two parental genomes. By careful phenotyping of each rat in the F2 generation, different phenotypic characteristics can be linked to specific genomic regions using microsatellite markers. In practice, a whole-genome search for susceptibility loci for a complex disease requires at least 200 F2 animals [44, 45].

Another approach to identify candidate genes is to analyze gene expression using techniques for differential display (reverse transcription-polymerase chain reaction), in order to detect RNA messages that are differentially regulated. Recent technical advances involving the use of gene chip technology allow studies in which levels of several thousand RNA messages can be simultaneously compared [46]. Both these approaches are very laborious, and a combination of the two may be needed to succeed in identifying the responsible genes. However, the perspective of pinpointing genes critically regulating glial reactivity, glial MHC expression and, even more so, mechanisms involved in nerve cell death certainly encourages further efforts in this direction. A hypothetical model for how different types of genes with impact on MS susceptibility may functionally interact is presented in Fig. 1.

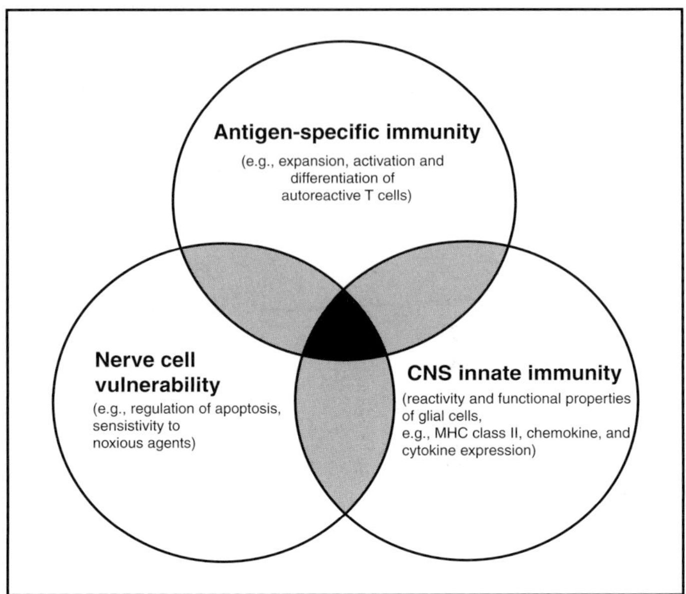

Fig. 1. Hypothetical model for how susceptibility genes for multiple sclerosis/experimental autoimmune encephalomyelitis (MS/EAE) can be categorized into different spheres depending on their function. Thus genes belonging to more than one of these groups may be needed for the development of clinical disease. The specific set of genes and from which spheres they are derived may also explain the large variability in symptoms and disease progression between different individuals suffering from MS

Trophic Interactions Between the Nervous and Immune Systems

One of the hallmarks of MS pathology is the accumulation of inflammatory cell infiltrates in the CNS parenchyma, and it is now widely accepted that leukocytes, and in particular CD4+ T cells, orchestrate the inflammatory assault directed to myelin sheaths. However, the role leukocytes may play in the progression of nerve cell damage and ultimately nerve cell death that accompanies white matter destruction remains unclear. The priority for resolving this question has increased considerably, since recent studies provide firm evidence that the degree of axonal destruction in MS plaques is a major correlate for permanent clinical disability [47-50]. It has generally been assumed to date that infiltration by activated leukocytes in the CNS and the ensuing inflammation have deleterious consequences for delicate neuronal networks, even if the exact mechanisms have remained unknown. In support of this notion, several studies have demonstrated that the highest degree of axonal damage occurs during the acute formation of plaques and that neuronal loss accompanies EAE [51-53]. So what is the role of leukocytes in these neurodegenerative processes? Experiments involving transfer of myelin protein-reactive and activated CD4+ T cells to naive recipients causes clinical EAE with typical histopathological damage to white matter tracts, which demonstrates their instrumental role in initiating disease [54, 55]. However, it is equally important to consider that autoimmune T cells can also be innocuous, as there are numerous examples of myelin peptide-reactive T cells that do not transfer disease. MS patients have increased numbers of myelin antigen-reactive T cells [56, 57], but of equal importance is that myelin protein-reactive T cells can also be cloned from healthy individuals and expand upon non-specific insults to the nervous system, such as viral infections [58], stroke [59], and peripheral nerve trauma [60, 61].

One of the most important biological questions in neuroimmunology that remains to be resolved is what are the characteristics that make an autoimmune T cell encephalitogenic. Activated T cells infiltrating the CNS during inflammatory relapses in MS or EAE are known to express high levels of the two pro-inflammatory cytokines IFN-γ and TNF-α, and a large body of evidence links these substances to processes that are known to be harmful to neurons. For example, the production of cell toxic compounds such as glutamate agonists [62, 63] and nitric oxide [64-67] is upregulated in microglia and astrocytes. There are also data suggesting that pro-inflammatory cytokines could have direct toxic effects on neurons [68, 69].

Paradoxically, a recent report demonstrated expression of the neuronal growth factor brain-derived neurotrophic factor (BDNF) in CNS infiltrating leukocytes in MS autopsy material [70]. BDNF belongs to the nerve growth factor (NGF) family of neuronal growth factors, which is also called the neurotrophin family. These factors are extremely important for the regulation of neuronal survival during development, but are also known to reduce neuronal loss or atrophy after axonal lesions in the adult [71-73]. Intriguingly, the expression of another neurotrophin family member, neurotrophin-3 (NT-3), together with BDNF was reported in human leukocyte populations [74]. With this as a background we wanted to explore whether CNS infiltrating leukocytes could enhance the survival of axotomized CNS neurons. For this purpose we used the VRA lesion paradigm alone or in combination with EAE induced by immunization with an encephalitogenic myelin basic protein peptide. Survival of motoneurons was assessed both during the peak of the disease and in the remission phase in two different rat strains. At all time points and in both strains the combination of VRA and EAE increased survival (50%-120%) compared with VRA alone [69]. As expected, very high levels of the pro-inflammatory cytokines IFN-γ and TNF-α were detected during the peak of the disease. More surprisingly, levels of BDNF and NT-3 were also highly induced in EAE animals. Characterization of neurotrophin expression in various leukocyte populations infiltrating the CNS demonstrated that levels of the substances were highly expressed in T cells and natural killer cells [69]. Although several mechanisms may be involved in the death of motoneurons in the VRA model, the fact that administration of BDNF strongly enhances neuronal survival after VRA [71, 75] demonstrates that deprivation of neuronal growth factors is one of the major determinants of cell death in this injury model. Furthermore, combined treatment of embryonic motoneuron cultures with IFN-γ or TNF-α and neurotrophins attenuated the death of cultured neurons treated with cytokines alone [69].

The notion that CNS infiltrating leukocytes are capable of supporting lesioned nerve cells is further supported by the observation that transfer of myelin autoreactive T cell lines to animals subjected to an optic nerve crush rescues a proportion of the lesioned retinal ganglion cells [76]. In fact, an overt immune reaction against CNS antigens may not be needed at all, since the loss of motoneurons after facial nerve transection in *scid* mice lacking functional T and B cells is aggravated compared with wildtype controls, an effect that can be blocked by reconstituting *scid* mice with wild type splenocytes [77]. Taken together, these results suggest that leukocytes recruited to the CNS may protect neurons from various harmful mediators generated by inflammatory processes in the CNS, and that the protective effect is mediated by the release of several different neurotrophic molecules (Fig. 2).

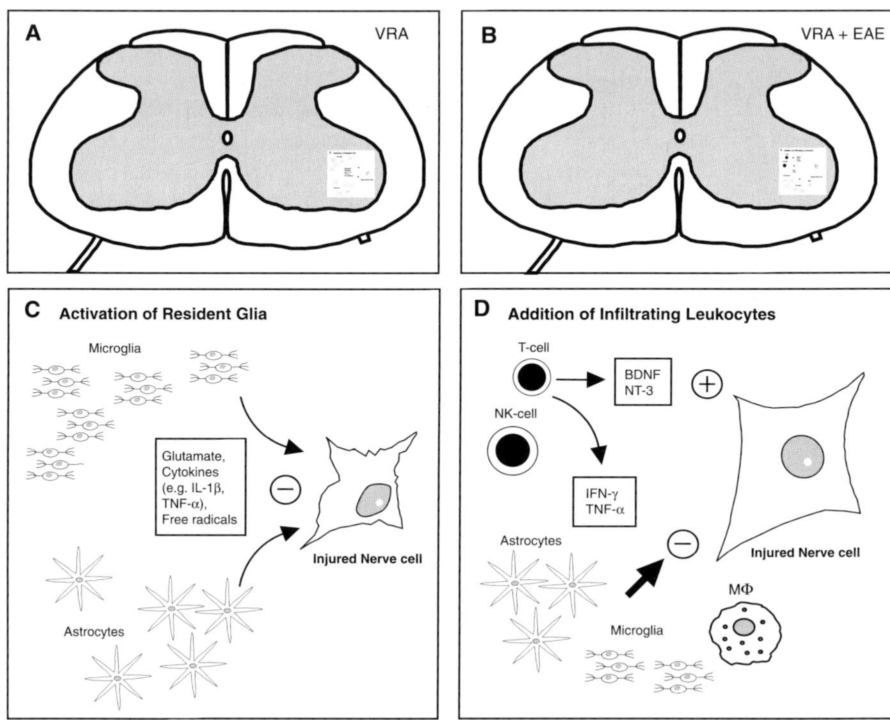

Fig. 2. Unilateral avulsion of ventral roots (VRA) leads to a retrograde reaction consisting of activation of surrounding glia and the subsequent death of a large proportion of the axotomized motoneurons (**A, B**). **C** The generation of neurotoxic compounds such as glutamate agonists, cytokines, and free radicals by the inflammatory reaction is likely to have negative consequences for the survival of lesioned neurons. **D** When VRA is combined with EAE the release of pro-inflammatory cytokines and chemokines from infiltrating leukocytes causes increased activation of resident glia and recruitment of macrophages (*MΦ*). This results in increased levels of neurotoxic substances (illustrated by a *thicker arrow* in **D**). In spite of this, both the degree of degeneration and atrophy of axotomized neurons are reduced (illustrated by a less atrophic nerve cell in **D**). Concomitant with the release of cytokines, infiltrating leukocytes, including encephalitogenic and bystander recruited T cells, as well as natural killer (NK) cells, express several neurotrophic factors, such as brain-derived neurohoptic factor (BDNF) and neurotrophin-3 (NT-3)

In some conditions, such as cerebrovascular diseases or mechanical nerve injuries, the influx of leukocytes (some of which may be CNS antigen reactive) at the site of the lesion may therefore be important for limiting the degree of neuronal loss. However, in MS/EAE the fact that leukocytes produce neurotrophic factors is even more intriguing, as there is evidence that these types of factors have immunomodulatory roles, for example by changing the cytokine profile of T helper cells, and that exogenous administration of NGF protects against EAE [78]. Future studies are therefore required to explore the possibility that neurotrophins may be used as therapeutic agents in MS or if it is possible to direct the functional characteristics of a T cell response from encephalitogenicity towards neuroprotection.

Acknowledgements. We thank Associate Professor Robert A. Harris for expert advice. This work was supported by Åke Wibergs, Magn Bergvalls, and Tore Nilsons stiftelse, NHR and the Swedish Medical Research Council, and the EU Biomed 2 Program (contract no. BMH4-97-202).

References

1. Risch N (1990) Linkage strategies for genetically complex traits. I. Multilocus models. Am J Hum Genet 46:222-228
2. Risch N (1990) Linkage strategies for genetically complex traits. II. The power of affected relative pairs. Am J Hum Genet 46:229-241
3. Risch N (1990) Linkage strategies for genetically complex traits. III. The effect of marker polymorphism on analysis of affected relative pairs [published erratum appears in Am J Hum Genet 1992 51:673-675]. Am J Hum Genet 46:242-253
4. Ebers GC, Bulman DE, Sadovnick AD et al (1986) A population-based study of multiple sclerosis in twins. N Engl J Med 315:1638-1642
5. Masterman T, Ligers A, Olsson T, Andersson M, Olerup O, Hillert J (2000) HLA-DR15 is associated with lower age at onset in multiple sclerosis. Ann Neurol 48:211-219
6. Marrosu MG, Murru MR, Costa G, Murru R, Muntoni F, Cucca F (1998) DRB1-DQA1-DQB1 loci and multiple sclerosis predisposition in the Sardinian population. Hum Mol Genet 7:1235-1237
7. Olerup O, Hillert J (1991) HLA class II-associated genetic susceptibility in multiple sclerosis: a critical evaluation. Tissue Antigens 38:1-15
8. Sawcer S, Jones H, Feakes R, Gray J, Smaldon N, Chataway J, Robertson N, Clayton D, Goodfellow P, Compston A (1996) A genome screen in multiple sclerosis reveals susceptibility loci on chromosome 6p21 and 17q22. Nat Genet 13:464-468
9. Haines JL, Ter-Minassian M, Bazyk A et al (1996) A complete genomic screen for multiple sclerosis underscores a role for the major histocompatability complex. The Multiple Sclerosis Genetics Group. Nat Genet 13:469-471
10. Ebers GC, Sadovnick AD (1994) The role of genetic factors in multiple sclerosis susceptibility. J Neuroimmunol 54:1-17
11. Haines JL, Terwedow HA, Burgess K, Pericak-Vance MA, Rimmler JB, Martin ER, Oksenberg JR, Lincoln R, Zhang DY, Banatao DR, Gatto N, Goodkin DE, Hauser SL (1998) Linkage of the MHC to familial multiple sclerosis suggests genetic heterogeneity. The Multiple Sclerosis Genetics Group. Hum Mol Genet 7:1229-1234

12. Weissert R, Wallström E, Storch M, Stefferl A, Lorentzen J, Lassmann H, Linington C, Olsson T (1998) MHC haplotype-dependent regulation of MOG-induced EAE in rats. J Clin Invest 102:1265-1273

13. Chataway J, Feakes R, Coraddu F, Gray J, Deans J, Fraser M, Robertson N, Broadley S, Jones H, Clayton D, Goodfellow P, Sawcer S, Compston A (1998) The genetics of multiple sclerosis: principles, background and updated results of the United Kingdom systematic genome screen. Brain 121:1869-1887

14. Lorentzen JC, Andersson M, Issazadeh S, Dahlman I, Luthman H, Weissert R, Olsson T (1997) Genetic analysis of inflammation, cytokine mRNA expression and disease course of relapsing experimental autoimmune encephalomyelitis in DA rats. J Neuroimmunol 80:31-37

15. Kjellén P, Issazadeh S, Olsson T, Holmdahl R (1998) Genetic influence on disease course and cytokine response in relapsing experimental allergic encephalomyelitis. Int Immunol 10:333-340

16. Roth MP, Viratelle C, Dolbois L, Delverdier M, Borot N, Pelletier L, Druet P, Clanet M, Coppin H (1999) A genome-wide search identifies two susceptibility loci for experimental autoimmune encephalomyelitis on rat chromosomes 4 and 10. J Immunol 162:1917-1922

17. Dahlman I, Lorentzen J, de Graaf K, Stefferl A, Linington C, Luthman H, Olsson T (1998) Quantitative trait loci disposing for both experimental arthritis and encephalomyelitis in the DA rat; impact on severity of myelin oligodendrocyte glycoprotein-induced experimental autoimmune encephalomyelitis and antibody isotype pattern. Eur J Immunol 28:2188-2196

18. Dahlman I, Wallstrom E, Weissert R, Storch M, Kornek B, Jacobsson L, Linington C, Luthman H, Lassmann H, Olsson T (1999) Linkage analysis of myelin oligodendrocyte glycoprotein-induced experimental autoimmune encephalomyelitis in the rat identifies a locus controlling demyelination on chromosome 18. Hum Mol Genet 8:2183-2190

19. Dahlman I, Jacobsson L, Lorentzen JC, Glaser A, Luthman H, Olsson T (1999) A genome wide linkage analysis of chronic relapsing experimental autoimmune encephalomyelitis in the rat identifies a major susceptibility locus on chromosome 9. J Immunol 162:2581-2588

20. Baker D, Butler D, Scallon BJ, O'Neill JK, Turk JL, Feldmann M (1994) Control of established experimental allergic encephalomyelitis by inhibition of tumor necrosis factor (TNF) activity within the central nervous system using monoclonal antibodies and TNF receptor-immunoglobulin fusion proteins. Eur J Immunol 24:2040-2048

21. Sundvall M, Jirholt J, Yang H, Jansson L, Engström A, Pettersson U, Holmdahl R (1995) Identification of murine loci associated with susceptibility to chronic experimental autoimmune encephalomyelitis. Nature Gen. 10:313-317

22. Encinas J, Lees M, Sobel R, Symonowicz C, Greer J, Shovlin CL, Weiner H, Seidman C, Seidman J, Kuchroo V (1996) Genetic analysis of susceptibility to experimental autoimmune encephalomyelitis in a cross between SJL/J and B10.S mice. J Immunol 157:2186-2192

23. Butterfield RJ, Sudweeks JD, Blankenhorn EP, Korngold R, Marini JC, Todd JA, Roper RJ, Teuscher C (1998) New genetic loci that control susceptibility and symptoms of experimental allergic encephalomyelitis in inbred mice. J Immunol 161:1860-1867

24. Becker KG, Simon RM, Bailey-Wilson JE, Freidlin B, Biddison WE, McFarland HF, Trent JM (1998) Clustering of non-major histocompatibility complex susceptibility candidate loci in human autoimmune diseases. Proc Natl Acad Sci USA 95:9979-9984

25. Vyse TJ, Todd JA (1996) Genetic analysis of autoimmune disease. Cell 85:311-318

26. Encinas JA, Wicker LS, Peterson LB, Mukasa A, Teuscher C, Sobel R, Weiner HL, Seidman CE, Seidman JG, Kuchroo VK (1999) QTL influencing autoimmune dia-

betes and encephalomyelitis map to a 0.15-cM region containing Il2 (letter). Nat Genet 21:158-160

27. van Walderveen MA, Barkhof F, Hommes OR, Polman CH, Tobi H, Frequin ST, Valk J (1995) Correlating MRI and clinical disease activity in multiple sclerosis: relevance of hypointense lesions on short-TR/short-TE (T1-weighted) spin-echo images. Neurology 45:1684-1690

28. Sedgwick JD, Schwender S, Gregersen R, Dorries R, ter Meulen V (1993) Resident macrophages (ramified microglia) of the adult brown Norway rat central nervous system are constitutively major histocompatibility complex class II positive. J Exp Med 177:1145-1152

29. Chung IY, Norris JG, Benveniste EN (1991) Differential tumor necrosis factor alpha expression by astrocytes from experimental allergic encephalomyelitis-susceptible and -resistant rat strains. J Exp Med 173:801-811

30. Linke A, Male D (1994) Strain-specific variation in constitutive and inducible expression of MHC class II, class I and ICAM-1 on rat cerebral endothelium. Immunology 82:88-94

31. Linke T, Greenwood J, Campbell I, Luthert P, Male DK (1998) Strain specific variation in IFN-gamma inducible lymphocyte adhesion to rat brain endothelial cells. J Neuroimmunol 91:28-32

32. Linke AT, Antonopoulos M, Davies DH, Male DK (2000) Strain specific variation in cytokine regulated ICAM-1 expression by rat brain-endothelial cells. J Neuroimmunol 104:10-14

33. Popovich PG, Wei P, Stokes BT (1997) Cellular inflammatory response after spinal cord injury in Sprague-Dawley and Lewis rats. J Comp Neurol 377:443-464

34. Kreutzberg GW, Graeber MB, Streit WJ (1989) Neuron-glial relationship during regeneration of motorneurons. Metab Brain Dis 4:81-85

35. Aldskogius H, Svensson M (1993) Neuronal and glial responses to axon injury. In: Malhotra SK (ed) Advances in structural biology. JAI Press, Greenwich, Connecticut, pp 191-223.

36. Maehlen J, Schroder H, Klareskog L, Olsson T, Kristensson K (1988) Axotomy induces MHC class I antigen expression on rat nerve cells. Neurosci Lett 92:8-13

37. Olsson T, Kristensson K, Ljungdahl A, Maehlen J, Holmdahl R, Klareskog L (1989) Gamma-interferon-like immunoreactivity in axotomized rat motor neurons. J Neurosci 9:3870-3875

38. Streit WJ, Graeber MB, Kreutzberg GW (1989) Expression of Ia antigen on perivascular and microglial cells after sublethal and lethal motor neuron injury. Exp Neurol 105:115-126

39. Koliatsos VE, Price WL, Pardo CA, Price DL (1994) Ventral root avulsion: an experimental model of death of adult motor neurons. J Comp Neurol 342:35-44

40. Piehl F, Tabar G, Cullheim S (1995) Expression of NMDA receptor mRNAs in rat motoneurons is down-regulated after axotomy. Eur J Neurosci 7:2101-2110

41. Piehl F, Lundberg C, Khademi M, Dahlman I, Lorentzen J, Olsson T (1999) Non-MHC gene regulation of nerve root injury-induced spinal cord inflammation and neuron death. J Neuroimmunol 101:87-97

42. Lorentzen JC, Issazadeh S, Storch M, Mustafa MI, Lassman H, Linington C, Klareskog L, Olsson T (1995) Protracted, relapsing and demyelinating experimental autoimmune encephalomyelitis in DA rats immunized with syngeneic spinal cord and incomplete Freund's adjuvant. J Neuroimmunol 63:193-205

43. Lundberg C, Lidman O, Holmdahl R, Olsson T, Piehl F (2001) Neurodegeneration and glial activation patterns after mechanical nerve injury are differentially regulated by non-MHC genes in congenic inbred rat strains. J Comp Neurol 431:75-87

44. Serikawa T, Kuramoto T, Hilbert P et al (1992) Rat gene mapping using PCR-analyzed microsatellites. Genetics 131:701-721

45. Olsson T, Dahlman I, Wallstrom E, Weissert R, Piehl F (2000) Genetics of rat neuroinflammation. J Neuroimmunol 107:191-200
46. Duggan DJ, Bittner M, Chen Y, Meltzer P, Trent JM (1999) Expression profiling using cDNA microarrays. Nat Genet 21:10-14
47. Davie CA, Barker GJ, Webb S, Tofts PS, Thompson AJ, Harding AE, McDonald WI, Miller DH (1995) Persistent functional deficit in multiple sclerosis and autosomal dominant cerebellar ataxia is associated with axon loss [published erratum appears in Brain 1996 119:1415]. Brain 118:1583-1592
48. De Stefano N, Matthews PM, Fu L, Narayanan S, Stanley J, Francis GS, Antel JP, Arnold DL (1998) Axonal damage correlates with disability in patients with relapsing-remitting multiple sclerosis. Results of a longitudinal magnetic resonance spectroscopy study. Brain 121:1469-1477
49. Lee MA, Blamire AM, Pendlebury S, Ho KH, Mills KR, Styles P, Palace J, Matthews PM (2000) Axonal injury or loss in the internal capsule and motor impairment in multiple sclerosis. Arch Neurol 57:65-70
50. Reddy H, Narayanan S, Matthews PM, Hoge RD, Pike GB, Duquette P, Antel J, Arnold DL (2000) Relating axonal injury to functional recovery in MS. Neurology 54:236-239
51. Ferguson B, Matyszak MK, Esiri MM, Perry VH (1997) Axonal damage in acute multiple sclerosis lesions. Brain 120:393-399
52. Trapp B, Peterson J, Ransohoff R, Rudick R, Mørk S, Bø L (1998) Axonal transection in the lesions of multiple sclerosis. N Engl J Med 338:278-285
53. Smith T, Groom A, Zhu B, Turski L (2000) Autoimmune encephalomyelitis ameliorated by AMPA antagonists. Nat Med 6:62-66
54. Ben-Nun A, Wekerle H, Cohen IR (1981) The rapid isolation of clonable antigen-specific T lymphocyte lines capable of mediating autoimmune encephalomyelitis. Eur J Immunol 11:195-199
55. Pettinelli CB, McFarlin DE (1981) Adoptive transfer of experimental allergic encephalomyelitis in SJL/J mice after in vitro activation of lymph node cells by myelin basic protein: requirement for Lyt 1+ 2− T lymphocytes. J Immunol 127:1420-1423
56. Olsson T, Zhi WW, Hojeberg B, Kostulas V, Jiang YP, Anderson G, Ekre HP, Link H (1990) Autoreactive T lymphocytes in multiple sclerosis determined by antigen-induced secretion of interferon-gamma. J Clin Invest 86:981-985
57. Zhang J, Medaer R, Stinissen P, Hafler D, Raus J (1993) MHC-restricted depletion of human myelin basic protein-reactive T cells by T cell vaccination. Science 261:1451-1454
58. Miller SD, Vanderlugt CL, Begolka WS, Pao W, Yauch RL, Neville KL, Katz-Levy Y, Carrizosa A, Kim BS (1997) Persistent infection with Theiler's virus leads to CNS autoimmunity via epitope spreading. Nat Med 3:1133-1136
59. Wang W, Olsson T, Kostulas V, Höjeberg B, Ekre H, Link H (1992) Myelin antigen reactive T cells in cerebrovascular diseases. Clin Exp Immunol 88:157-162
60. Olsson T, Diener P, Ljungdahl Å, Höjeberg B, van der Meide P, Kristensson K (1992) Facial nerve transection causes expansion of myelin autoreactive T cells in regional lymph nodes and T cell homing to the facial nucleus. Autoimmunity 13:117-126
61. Olsson T, Sun JB, Solders G, Xiao BG, Höjeberg B, Ekre HP, Link H (1993) Autoreactive T and B cell responses to myelin antigens after diagnostic sural nerve biopsy. J Neurol Sci 117:130-139
62. Piani D, Spranger M, Frei K, Schaffner A, Fontana A (1992) Macrophage-induced cytotoxicity of N-methyl-D-aspartate receptor positive neurons involves excitatory amino acids rather than reactive oxygen intermediates and cytokines. Eur J Immunol 22:2429-2436
63. Giulian D, Corpuz M, Chapman S, Mansouri M, Robertson C (1993) Reactive mononuclear phagocytes release neurotoxins after ischemic and traumatic injury to the central nervous system. J Neurosci Res 36:681-693

64. Chao C, Hu S, Molitor T, Shaskan E, Peterson P (1992) Activated microglia mediate neuronal cell injury via a nitric oxide mechanism. J Immunol 149:2736-2741
65. Chao CC, Hu S, Ehrlich L, Peterson PK (1995) Interleukin-1 and tumor necrosis factor-alpha synergistically mediate neurotoxicity: involvement of nitric oxide and of *N*-methyl-D-aspartate receptors. Brain Behav Immun 9:355-365
66. Lee SC, Dickson DW, Liu W, Brosnan CF (1993) Induction of nitric oxide synthase activity in human astrocytes by interleukin-1 beta and interferon-gamma. J Neuroimmunol 46:19-24
67. Merrill JE, Ignarro LJ, Sherman MP, Melinek J, Lane TE (1993) Microglial cell cytotoxicity of oligodendrocytes is mediated through nitric oxide. J Immunol 151:2132-2141
68. Talley AK, Dewhurst S, Perry SW, Dollard SC, Gummuluru S, Fine SM, New D, Epstein LG, Gendelman HE, Gelbard HA (1995) Tumor necrosis factor alpha-induced apoptosis in human neuronal cells: protection by the antioxidant *N*-acetyl-cysteine and the genes *bcl-2* and *crmA*. Mol Cell Biol 15:2359-2366
69. Hammarberg H, Lidman O, Lundberg C, Eltayeb SY, Gielen AW, Muhallab S, Svenningsson A, Linda H, van der Meide PH, Cullheim S, Olsson T, Piehl F (2000) Neuroprotection by encephalomyelitis: rescue of mechanically injured neurons and neurotrophin production by CNS-infiltrating T and natural killer cells. J Neurosci 20:5283-5291
70. Kerschensteiner M, Gallmeier E, Behrens L, Leal VV, Misgeld T, Klinkert WE, Kolbeck R, Hoppe E, Oropeza-Wekerle RL, Bartke I, Stadelmann C, Lassmann H, Wekerle H, Hohlfeld R (1999) Activated human T cells, B cells, and monocytes produce brain-derived neurotrophic factor in vitro and in inflammatory brain lesions: a neuroprotective role of inflammation? J Exp Med 189:865-870
71. Kishino A, Ishige Y, Tatsuno T, Nakayama C, Noguchi H (1997) BDNF prevents and reverses adult rat motor neuron degeneration and induces axonal outgrowth. Exp Neurol 144:273-286
72. Kobayashi NR, Fan DP, Giehl KM, Bedard AM, Wiegand SJ, Tetzlaff W (1997) BDNF and NT-4/5 prevent atrophy of rat rubrospinal neurons after cervical axotomy, stimulate GAP-43 and Talpha1-tubulin mRNA expression, and promote axonal regeneration. J Neurosci 17:9583-9595
73. Hammond EN, Tetzlaff W, Mestres P, Giehl KM (1999) BDNF, but not NT-3, promotes long-term survival of axotomized adult rat corticospinal neurons in vivo. Neuroreport 10:2671-2675
74. Besser M, Wank R (1999) Cutting edge: clonally restricted production of the neurotrophins brain-derived neurotrophic factor and neurotrophin-3 mRNA by human immune cells and Th1/Th2-polarized expression of their receptors. J Immunol 162:6303-6306
75. Novikov L, Novikova L, Kellerth JO (1995) Brain-derived neurotrophic factor promotes survival and blocks nitric oxide synthase expression in adult rat spinal motoneurons after ventral root avulsion. Neurosci Lett 200:45-48
76. Moalem G, Leibowitz-Amit R, Yoles E, Mor F, Cohen I, Schwartz M (1999) Autoimmune T cells protect neurons from secondary degeneration after central nervous system axotomy. Nat Med 5:49-55
77. Serpe C, Kohm A, Huppenbauer C, Sanders V, Jones K (1999) Exacerbation of facial motoneuron loss after facial nerve transection in severe combined immunodeficient (scid) mice. J Neurosci 19:RC7
78. Villoslada P, Hauser SL, Bartke I, Unger J, Heald N, Rosenberg D, Cheung SW, Mobley WC, Fisher S, Genain CP (2000) Human nerve growth factor protects common marmosets against autoimmune encephalomyelitis by switching the balance of T helper cell type 1 and 2 cytokines within the central nervous system. J Exp Med 191:1799-1806

Neuroprotective Treatment in Primary Progressive Multiple Sclerosis: a Phase I/II Study with Riluzole

N. KALKERS, F. BARKHOF, L. BERGERS, R. VAN SCHIJNDEL, C. POLMAN

Introduction

Most currently available treatments for multiple sclerosis (MS), in particular corticosteroids and interferon β, especially address the inflammatory component of the disease. Their main clinical impact is on relapses whereas an effect on permanent disability so far has been less well established. This might be explained by observations, especially from magnetic resonance imaging (MRI) studies, that the correlation of inflammation with disease progression and development of disability is poor [1].

Recent evidence suggests that axonal loss may occur more early in the disease course of MS than previously anticipated; most likely it is the pathological correlate of irreversible neurological impairment. Ferguson et al. [2] found large numbers of damaged axons in acute lesions and at the border of chronic active lesions, but not in chronic lesions. Trapp et al. [3] observed abundant axonal transection in active and chronic active lesions from patients whose clinical disease duration ranged from weeks to 27 years. Magnetic resonance spectroscopy studies measuring N-acetylaspartate, a marker of axonal damage, suggest that axonal damage or loss occurs both in lesions and in normal-appearing white matter, and that it begins in the early stages of MS and may contribute to chronic disability [4-6]. These observations support the pursuit of neuroprotective therapeutic strategies in MS, as recommended in authoritative editorials [7, 8].

Here we present the results of a pilot study investigating the effects of the neuroprotective agent riluzole in primary progressive (PP) MS patients. This group of MS patients shows less inflammatory activity, a reason why they are typically excluded from clinical trials. Riluzole is an approved treatment for amyotrophic lateral sclerosis (ALS); it has been shown to provide a greater probability of survival in patients suffering from this disease [9]. The drug appears to act through inhibition of glutamate transmission in the central nervous system (CNS). Glutamate acts as an excitotoxin, participating in the process of neuronal damage.

Recent MRI studies suggest that T1-hypointense lesions ('black holes') and atrophy of brain and spinal cord are imaging correlates of axonal loss [10]. A number of groups have also reported that atrophy develops early in the disease course and correlates more strongly with clinical progression than other MRI changes like T2-lesions or gadolinium enhancement [11-16]. These measurements have therefore been proposed as potentially suitable outcome parameters for the evaluation of therapeutic efficacy in PPMS, and were used in this study [17].

Patients and Methods

Patients

The study patients, all of whom were aged between 18 and 70 years, had PPMS with documented progression during the 24 months before inclusion. Kurtzke's Expanded Disability Status Scale (EDSS) scores were between 3.0 (inclusive) and 7.5 (inclusive) [18]. Recipients of immunomodulatory drugs and patients with other medical or systemic diseases that might interfere with assessment of disability were excluded. Women of childbearing potential who were pregnant, nursing, or not using adequate birth control measures were also excluded.

Design

The study was approved by the hospital ethics committee and after providing informed consent, 16 patients were selected from a natural history cohort of PPMS. The study duration was 24 months. During the first 12 months no specific treatment was given and during the second 12 months all patients were treated with riluzole (2 × 50 mg daily). At entry into the trial, demographic data were obtained, a full history taken, and a neurological examination performed. Patients underwent further examinations after 6, 12, 18, and 24 months. At each visit, extensive MRI investigations and a short physical examination were performed, and EDSS scores were obtained at 0, 12, and 24 months. MRI included magnetization prepared rapid acquisition gradient echo (MPRAGE) imaging at all visits, and T1- and T2-weighted sequences at 0, 12 and 24 months. Images were obtained at 1.0 T (Magnetom Impact, Siemens, Erlangen, Germany). All adverse events were documented; laboratory investigation included serum transaminases (monthly for 3 months and every 3 months thereafter) and hematology (complete blood count and differential every 6 months) after the start of treatment.

Analysis

The efficacy of riluzole was assessed by comparing mean change for spinal cord measurement and median changes for T1 and T2 lesion load measurements during the first 12 months of the study (without treatment) with those in the second 12 months (during treatment). The advantage of this analysis for a small pilot study is that it excludes inter-patient variability as an important confounding factor.

The primary outcome criterion selected was the change in spinal cord cross-sectional area between the 1-year periods. To obtain this information, a series of ten contiguous 3-mm axial slices from the MPRAGE data set were reformatted perpendicular to the cord above the center of the C2-C3 disc. A blinded observer reformatted all slices twice (Radworks 4.0, Applicare Medical Imaging, Alphen ad Rijn, The Netherlands) and scored the spinal cord area (in mm^2), with a homemade semi-automated, local thresholding, seed-growing method. The coefficient of variation for this method in our hands was 1.3%. The mean of these two measurements was used for further analysis. Scans were analyzed serially, although in a randomized and blinded fashion. Secondary outcome criteria defined were the total unenhanced T1 lesion volume ('black holes'), the total T2 lesion volume, and the number of gadolinium-enhancing lesions on brain MRI, as well as the EDSS.

Safety data were evaluated for all patients treated, efficacy data only for those patients who continued treatment for at least 3 months, for which we used all available data.

Statistics

Mean and median results were calculated, as well as median increase per year of all evaluable scans, expressed as percentages. Student's *t*-test for normally distributed data (MPRAGE and EDSS) and Wilcoxon test for non-parametric data (T1 and T2 lesion load, gadolinium-enhancing lesions) were used to evaluate the difference between the year without treatment and the year on treatment.

Results

Patient demographics and clinical data are presented in Table 1.

Two patients discontinued treatment because of side effects (1 patient after about 1 month because of headache, 1 patient after 2 months because of increase in spasticity, reduction in muscle strength, and fatigue). Five patients needed intermittent reduction in dosage of study drug (3 because of reduced muscle strength, increase in spasticity, and balance disorders causing mobility problems, 2 because of sensory disturbances and increased fatigue). In 14 patients who took medication for over 3 months, medically severe adverse effects were not observed.

Table 1. Demographic and clinical data [medians (range)]

Number	Sex (F:M)	Age (years)	Duration of symptoms (years)	EDSS t=0
16	9:7	51.5 (30-66)	9.5 (2.9-32.3)	6.0 (3.5-7.5)

Table 2. Results on primary and secondary magnetic resonance imaging (MRI) outcome parameters

MRI parameter	Baseline	1-year	2-year	Change during 1st year[c] (without treatment)	Change during 2nd year[c] (with treatment)
Spinal cord area[a]	66.7 (9.1)	65.4	65.2	−2.0%	−0.2%
T1 lesion load[b]	271 (0-7,032)	403 (0-9,393)	369 (129-9,243)	+15%	+6%
T2 lesion load[b]	2,160 (513-3,2892)	3,343 (540-28,008)	4,206 (600-28,800)	+7.0%	+10%

[a] Mean, mm^2 (SD)
[b] Median, mm^3 (range)
[c] Median change of all evaluable scans

For MPRAGE analysis we had to exclude 1 patient, first because of missing baseline data (due to a wrong scan protocol) and secondly because of insufficient quality of follow-up scans (due to technical problems). For the remaining 13 patients (65 scans), an additional 5 scans could not be quantified for the primary outcome criterion due to technical problems or poor quality of scans (difficulty in adhering to extensive MRI protocol; movement artefacts). For quantification of T1- and T2- weighted imaging, 2 baseline scans were missing (1 due to a wrong scan protocol and 1 due to technical problems). Table 2 presents the mean spinal cord area at all time points, analyzed including all available data for all patients. There is a reduction of mean spinal cord area in the 1st year (2%) and a trend for stabilization in the 2nd year (0.2%, Fig. 1); this trend, however, was not statistically significant. The secondary outcome parameters, T1 and T2 lesion loads, both increased during the study (Table 2). Whereas the increase in T2 lesion load was essentially the same or even tended to accelerate during the 1st and 2nd year (increase of 7% and 10%, respectively), there was a trend, although not statistically significant, for the increase in T1 lesion load to be reduced during the 2nd year of the study (15 versus 6%, respectively). The median number of gadolinium lesions was 0 at all time points. The median EDSS changed in the 1st year of the study from 6.0 to 6.5; the median EDSS remained 6.5 at 24 months.

Discussion

The results from this pilot study, as far as we know the first of neuroprotective treatment in MS, suggest an effect on MRI parameters of axonal loss during 12 months of treatment with riluzole, although this effect did not reach levels of statistical significance.

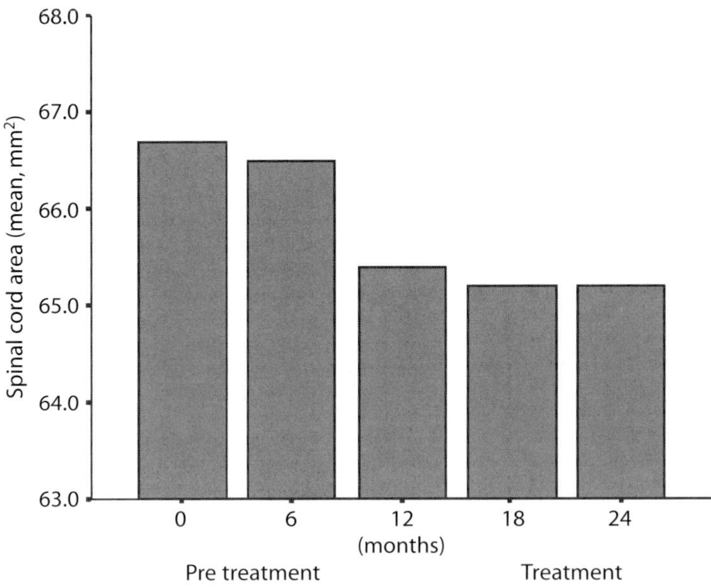

Fig. 1. Spinal cord area (mean, mm²) months 0 - 12 without treatment and months 12 - 24 with treatment

Spinal cord atrophy is a relatively new outcome parameter in MS clinical trials. It has been validated by studies that have shown a good correlation between spinal cord atrophy and disability in MS [11, 15] and by a longitudinal study that showed that it was possible to measure changes in cord cross-sectional area over time, especially in patients with PPMS [17]. In this last study the reduction in cord size was about 5% over a 1-year period in PPMS patients, which seems to be somewhat larger than the 2% we observed during the 1 year of our study. Since the techniques applied in both studies are very similar, we assume that this difference can be accounted for by differences in patient selection. Based on a comparison of these studies it probably is safe to conclude that the difference in development of atrophy that was observed between the 1st and the 2nd year in our study was not due to an excessive change during the 1st year. We also found a dissociation of the effects of riluzole on T1 and T2 lesion load. There was a clear trend for reduced increase of T1 lesion load during treatment (median increase of 15 % in 1st and 6% in 2nd year of study) in the absence of a reduced increase in T2 lesion load (median increase 7% in 1st and 10% in 2nd year). Whereas T2 lesion load is non-specific and reflects the total lesion load in MS, recent studies, applying both pathological examination of autopsy and biopsy material as well as in vivo magnetic resonance spectroscopy, have clearly shown that hypointense areas on T1-weighted imaging strongly correlate with the destructive character of lesions, more specifically axonal loss [5, 10, 19, 20]. Remarkably, another recently published study, applying novel MRI techniques in monitoring the effect of treatment on the pathological process in MS, found the same dissociation, although in the opposite direction. Treatment with the lymphocyte-depleting humanized monoclonal antibody Campath 1H strongly reduced the number of new inflammatory lesions, although it had no effect on progression of atrophy and T1 lesion load [21, 22].

A recent study discusses the application of glutamate receptor blockade in an animal model of MS. Reduction of axonal damage was shown in experimental allergic encephalomyelitis, using the AMPA/ainate antagonist NBQX [23]. NBQX blocks the excitatory glutamate receptor of the oligodendrocytes and thereby, like riluzole, modulates glutaminergic transmission. Our observations are in line with the hypothesis that riluzole does not affect new lesion genesis, but as a neuroprotective agent does have an impact on subsequent lesion development, resulting in reduced axonal loss. It suggests an effect on MRI parameters of axonal loss, and provides the first human correlate of the observations by Pitt et al. [23], that glutamate excitotoxicity contributes to lesion development in demyelinating disease and therefore should be considered as an important therapeutic target. Of course our study does not allow an in-depth assessment of the potential value of riluzole in MS. Given the small sample size and the short duration of this study, as well as the possibility of 'regression to the mean', we recommend that additional data be obtained in a large placebo-controlled trial using a parallel-group design. The MRI characteristics observed in our study suggest that neuroprotective agents could be used for combination therapy with anti-inflammatory agents in MS.

References

1. Kappos L, Moeri D, Radue EW, Schoetzau A, Schweikert K, Barkhof F et al (1999) Predictive value of gadolinium-enhanced magnetic resonance imaging for relapse rate and changes in disability or impairment in multiple sclerosis: a meta-analysis. Gadolinium MRI Meta-analysis Group. Lancet 353:964-969
2. Ferguson B, Matyszak MK, Esiri MM, Perry VH (1997) Axonal damage in acute multiple sclerosis lesions. Brain 120:393-399
3. Trapp BD, Peterson J, Ransohoff RM, Rudick R, Mork S, Bo L (1998) Axonal transection in the lesions of multiple sclerosis. N Engl J Med 338:278-285
4. Fu L, Matthews PM, De Stefano N, Worsley KJ, Narayanan S, Francis GS et al (1998) Imaging axonal damage of normal-appearing white matter in multiple sclerosis. Brain 121:103-113
5. van Walderveen MA, Barkhof F, Pouwels PJ, van Schijndel RA, Polman CH, Castelijns JA (1999) Neuronal damage in T1-hypointense multiple sclerosis lesions demonstrated in vivo using proton magnetic resonance spectroscopy. Ann Neurol 46:79-87
6. De Stefano N, Narayanan S, Francis GS, Arnaoutelis R, Tartaglia MC, Antel JP et al (2001) Evidence of axonal damage in the early stages of multiple sclerosis and its relevance to disability. Arch Neurol 58:65-70
7. Scolding N, Franklin R (1998) Axon loss in multiple sclerosis. Lancet 352:340-341
8. Waxman SG (1998) Demyelinating diseases-new pathological insights, new therapeutic targets. N Engl J Med 338:323-325

9. Bensimon G, Lacomblez L, Meininger V, ALS/Riluzole Study Group (1994) A controlled trial of riluzole in amyotrophic lateral sclerosis. N Engl J Med 330:585-591
10. van Waesberghe JH, Kamphorst W, De Groot CJ, van Walderveen MA, Castelijns JA, Ravid R et al (1999) Axonal loss in multiple sclerosis lesions: magnetic resonance imaging insights into substrates of disability. Ann Neurol 46:747-754
11. Losseff NA, Webb SL, O'Riordan JI, Page R, Wang L, Barker GJ et al (1996) Spinal cord atrophy and disability in multiple sclerosis. A new reproducible and sensitive MRI method with potential to monitor disease progression. Brain 119:701-708
12. Losseff NA, Wang L, Lai HM, Yoo DS, Gawne-Cain ML, Mcdonald WI et al (1996) Progressive cerebral atrophy in multiple sclerosis. A serial MRI study. Brain 119:2009-2019
13. Edwards SG, Gong QY, Liu C, Zvartau ME, Jaspan T, Roberts N et al (1999) Infratentorial atrophy on magnetic resonance imaging and disability in multiple sclerosis. Brain 122:291-301
14. Rudick RA, Fisher E, Lee JC, Simon J, Jacobs L (1999) Use of the brain parenchymal fraction to measure whole brain atrophy in relapsing-remitting MS. Multiple Sclerosis Collaborative Research Group. Neurology 53(8):1698-1704
15. Nijeholt GJ, van Walderveen MA, Castelijns JA, van Waesberghe JH, Polman C, Scheltens P et al (1998) Brain and spinal cord abnormalities in multiple sclerosis. Correlation between MRI parameters, clinical subtypes and symptoms. Brain 121:687-697
16. Simon JH, Jacobs LD, Campion MK, Rudick RA, Cookfair DL, Herndon RM et al (1999) A longitudinal study of brain atrophy in relapsing multiple sclerosis. Neurology 53:139-148
17. Stevenson VL, Leary SM, Losseff NA, Parker GJ, Barker GJ, Husmani Y et al (1998) Spinal cord atrophy and disability in MS: a longitudinal study. Neurology 51:234-238
18. Kurtzke JF (1983) Rating neurologic impairment in multiple sclerosis: an expanded disability status scale (EDSS). Neurology 33:1444-1452
19. Bruck W, Bitsch A, Kolenda H, Bruck Y, Stiefel M, Lassmann H (1997) Inflammatory central nervous system demyelination: correlation of magnetic resonance imaging findings with lesion pathology. Ann Neurol 42:783-793
20. van Walderveen MA, Kamphorst W, Scheltens P, van Waesberghe JH, Ravid R, Valk J et al (1998) Histopathologic correlate of hypointense lesions on T1-weighted spin-echo MRI in multiple sclerosis. Neurology 50:1282-1288
21. Paolillo A, Coles AJ, Molyneux PD, Gawne-Cain M, MacManus D, Barker GJ et al (1999) Quantitative MRI in patients with secondary progressive MS treated with monoclonal antibody Campath 1H. Neurology 53:751-757
22. Coles AJ, Wing MG, Molyneux P, Paolillo A, Davie CM, Hale G et al (1999) Monoclonal antibody treatment exposes three mechanisms underlying the clinical course of multiple sclerosis. Ann Neurol 46:296-304
23. Pitt D, Werner P, Raine CS (2000) Glutamate excitotoxicity in a model of multiple sclerosis. Nat Med 6:67-70

Chapter 5

Neuropathology and Disease Progression in Multiple Sclerosis

C. BJARTMAR, B.D. TRAPP

Introduction

The histopathology of multiple sclerosis (MS) is characterized by focal inflammation, demyelination, loss of oligodendrocytes, reactive astrogliosis, and axonal pathology. Of these hallmarks, myelin loss has attracted most interest, and MS research has historically focused on mechanisms associated with inflammatory demyelination and remyelination. Although the neuropathology of MS is primarily demyelinating, a number of reports describe axonal injury in the disease [1-9]. In fact, axonal pathology in MS lesions was described more than a century ago [10]. Charcot (1868), for example, discussed MS lesions in terms of demyelination and astrogliosis, but he also mentioned axonal loss [11]. Current data on axonal pathology in MS have been provided through a variety of approaches, including magnetic resonance imaging (MRI) [7, 12-14], magnetic resonance spectroscopy (MRS) [2, 3, 5, 15] and morphological analysis of brain sections [4, 9]. Immunohistochemical studies have recently emphasized the correlation between inflammation and axonal damage during the early stages of MS [4, 9]. In addition, long-term axonal pathology has been described in a number of myelin protein gene knockout and transgenic mice models [6, 8, 16], as well as in chronic MS patients [17, 18], indicating that lack of myelin-related molecules can result in axonal pathology. Together, these data suggest that cumulative axonal degeneration constitutes a significant pathogenic component of MS, and indicate that loss of axons may be a main determinant of the progressive neurological disability seen in these patients [1, 3, 5, 6, 8, 17].

Axonal Injury During Early Stages of MS

Axonal transection occurs in cerebral MS lesions undergoing inflammatory demyelination [4, 9]. Ferguson et al. [9] demonstrated axonal amyloid precursor protein (APP) in active lesions and at the border of chronic active lesions. Accumulation of APP is considered a marker for axonal dysfunction and injury, since it is detected immunohistochemically only in axons with impaired axonal transport [19]. Many APP-immunoreactive structures resembled axonal ovoids, characteristic of newly transected axons. These results suggested axonal dysfunction within inflammatory MS lesions and indicated that many of these axons were undergoing transection.

These findings were confirmed and extended by a morphological investigation on lesions from MS brains with various degree of inflammation and disease durations from 2 weeks to 27 years [4]. Axonal ovoids were identified through three-dimensional confocal microscopy as terminal ends of transected axons immunostained for non-phosphorylated neurofilaments. The density of transected axons was over 11,000 mm^3 in active lesions and over 3,000 mm^3 at the edge of chronic active lesions. The core of chronic active lesions contained on average 875 transected axons per mm^3. In contrast, less than 1 axonal ovoid was detected per mm^3 in control white matter. Together, these data demonstrate a positive correlation between axonal transection and degree of inflammation in cerebral MS lesions undergoing demyelination. The presence of terminal ends in patients with short disease duration suggests that axonal transection begins at an early stage of MS [4].

The pathophysiology of axonal damage during early stages of MS is unknown, and we can only speculate on possible mechanisms. Since the extent of axonal damage in active MS lesions correlates with the inflammatory activity of the lesions [4, 9], axonal injury could be associated with the inflammation *per se* (Fig. 1). Inflammatory substances such as proteolytic

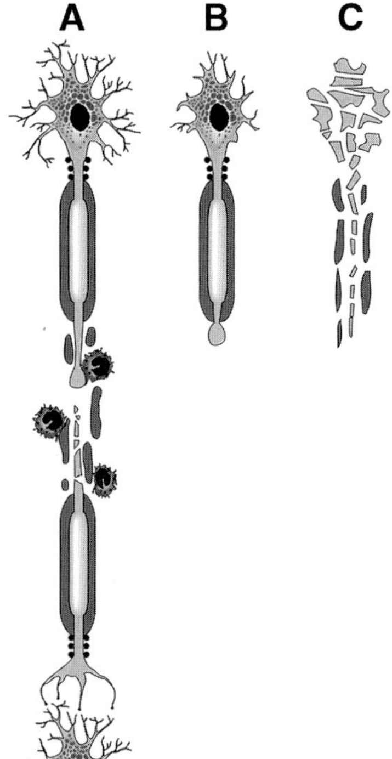

Fig. 1. Axonal transection during inflammatory demyelination (**A**) causes irreversible loss of neuronal function, denervation of target cells, and induces formation of terminal axonal ovoids. The distal axonal segment undergoes Wallerian degeneration (**B**) and retrograde neuronal Wallerian degeneration (**C**) may occur. During early stages of multiple sclerosis (MS), the CNS compensates for loss of axons. From [74]

enzymes, cytokines, oxidative products, and free radicals produced by activated immune and glial cells are potential mediators of such damage [20]. It is also possible that increased extracellular pressure caused by inflammatory edema can injure axons, particularly in the spinal cord where the space for tissue expansion is more limited than in the brain. Finally, since interactions between multiple genes most likely influence the outcome of MS in individual patients [21-23], it is possible that genes involved in axonal responses to inflammation and demyelination influence the extent of axonal damage and loss in MS [23-25].

Cumulative Axonal Loss in Long-Term MS

The presence of early axonal transection in MS, in the absence of obvious progressive disability between relapses, raises questions regarding the extent of long-term axonal loss during chronic disease. In order to quantify total axonal loss in MS lesions, an axonal sampling protocol that accounts for both tissue atrophy and reduced axonal density was developed using spinal cord cross sections [17]. Using this protocol, total axonal loss was quantified in 10 chronic inactive lesions from five MS patients with significant functional impairment (EDSS ≥7.5) and long disease duration. The lesions contained an average 68% (45%-84%) loss of axons compared with controls. These results demonstrate that axonal loss constitutes a significant part of the long-term pathology that develops in many chronic MS lesions (Fig. 2). Given the severe permanent neu-

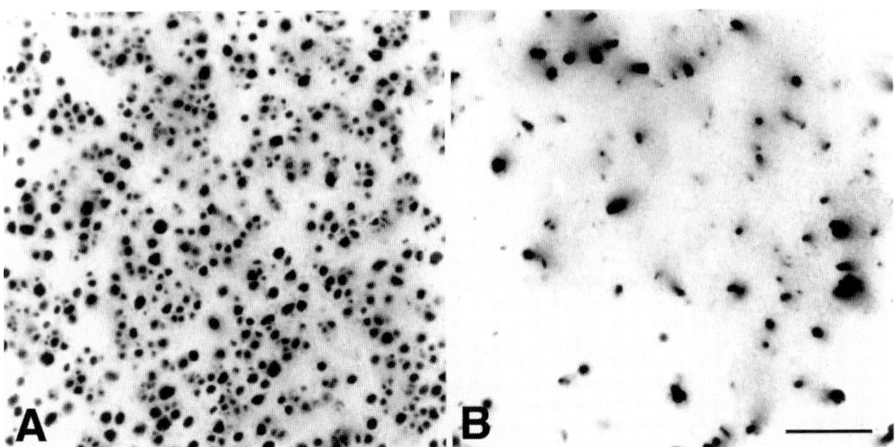

Fig. 2. Loss of axons in the spinal cord of a paralyzed patient with MS for 22 years. Neurofilament staining demonstrates axonal density in control (**A**) and in a demyelinated area in the gracile fasciculus of MS cervical spinal cord (**B**). This chronic inactive lesion exhibits severe axonal loss. Scale bar = 25 μm. From [6]

rological disability of the examined patients, the data also support axonal degeneration as the main cause of irreversible neurological disability in non-ambulatory MS patients. Average axonal density (number of axons per unit area) in these lesions was decreased by 58%. A similar reduction in axonal density, 61%, was recently reported in spinal cord lesions from patients with secondary progressive MS (SPMS) [18].

The extent of axonal loss in severely disabled patients with long disease duration, often without signs of inflammatory activity at later stages of disease, suggests that mechanisms other than inflammatory demyelination contribute to axonal transection in chronic MS lesions [17, 18]. A number of genes coding for myelin related proteins such as MAG, PLP, PMP22, P0 and connexin 32, contribute to the long-term viability of axons [26-30]. For example, late-onset axonal pathology such as atrophy or swelling, cytoskeleton alterations, organelle accumulation and degeneration was reported in mice lacking MAG [28] and PLP [29]. The axonal pathology in these mice was accompanied by progressive clinical disability, including impaired gait, tremor, and spasticity. Hence, chronically demyelinated axons may undergo degeneration due to lack of trophic support from myelin or oligodendrocytes (Fig. 3) [6, 8, 16].

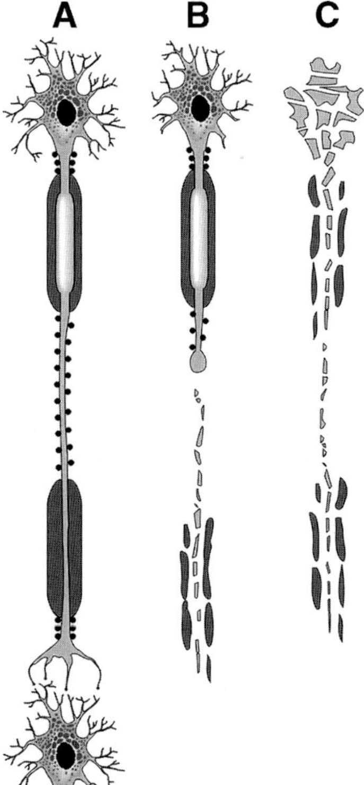

Fig. 3. Long-term axonal degeneration as a consequence of chronic demyelination (**A**). Myelin-derived factors have a trophic effect on axons. The lack of trophic support may cause axonal transection and Wallerian degeneration distally (**B**) or retrograde neuronal death (**C**). This mechanism of axonal loss may cause progressive functional decline during secondary progressive MS when inflammatory activity is reduced. From [74]

Axonal Degeneration in Non-Lesion MS White Matter

Transected central nervous system (CNS) axons will undergo relatively rapid Wallerian degeneration distal to the site of transection. In contrast, CNS myelin can persist for a long time after proximal fiber transection. Histologically, such remaining myelin sheaths will form empty tubes, or later degenerating ovoids. The white matter, however, may appear normal on conventional MRI. Recently, a number of postmortem studies have addressed the extent of axonal loss quantitatively in normal-appearing white matter. Lovas et al. [18] examined axonal density in lesions and in normal-appearing white matter from the cervical spinal cord of patients with SPMS. The decrease in axonal density in normal-appearing white matter was as much as 57%. Ganter et al. [31] reported reductions in axonal density of 19%-42% in the lateral corticospinal tract of MS patients with lower limb weakness. A study that accounted for both changes in tissue volume and decreased axonal density examined total axonal loss in MS patients with disease duration between 5 and 34 years and various degrees of functional impairment [32]. The average axonal loss in normal-appearing corpus callosum of these patients was 53%. Since the reduction in axonal density in the same material was only 34%, the data demonstrate that measures of both tissue volume and axonal density are necessary to determine total axonal loss. Together, these studies suggest that normal-appearing white matter, as seen on MRI scans or after immunohistochemistry for myelin, might contain considerable axonal loss, especially in chronic patients with long disease duration.

Neurodegeneration and Tissue Atrophy

Several MRI studies have suggested a correlation between clinical disability and atrophy of the cerebellum [12], spinal cord [13], and cerebral tissue [14] in MS. The correlation between atrophy and progressive functional impairment has been interpreted as a reflection of axonal loss. Since measurements of CNS atrophy may be used as a surrogate marker for disease progression in these patients, such correlation has significant clinical interest. It is generally accepted that total brain lesion volume, as measured on T2-weighted MRI scans, has low pathological specificity and poor correlation with clinical disability [33]. Motor performance has a relatively high impact on measurements of clinical disability in MS, such as EDSS. The spinal cord is therefore considered a suitable model to study the relationship between tissue atrophy and clinical progression. A number of reports indicate that spinal cord atrophy, as revealed by MRI, can correlate with clinical disability in MS [13, 34, 35]. In SPMS patients, cervical spinal cord atrophy averages 25%-30% [13, 17]. Spinal cord atrophy generally appears to be more pronounced in the cervical than in the lumbar cord [34].

The periventricular white matter is frequently affected by MS lesions, which might explain the progressive enlargement of lateral ventricles observed in many MS patients [8, 36, 37]. The degree of cerebral atrophy correlates with the degree of functional decline [14] and begins at an early stage of MS. In a group of relapsing-remitting MS (RRMS) patients with mild-to-moderate disability followed over 2 years, brain atrophy increased yearly [37, 38]. The course of brain atrophy appears to be influenced by general inflammatory disease activity, as indicated by the occurrence of gadolinium-enhanced lesions in these brains. A new sensitive measure of whole-brain atrophy was applied to this population of relapsing patients [38]. The brain parenchymal fraction (BPF), which constitutes the ratio of brain parenchyma to the total volume within the brain surface contour, was highly reproducible, thus allowing precise comparison of individual brain volumes. The BPF declined at a highly significant rate and was significantly reduced compared with age- and sex-matched control individuals during each of 2 years follow-up of these patients.

Axonal loss is a plausible contributor to atrophy in MS, although demyelination and reduced axon diameter may also decrease tissue volume [33]. However, many chronic MS lesions develop prominent astrogliosis [1, 17]. To what extent astrogliosis in MS lesions affects tissue atrophy remains to be determined. In chronic MS patients, the proportion of white to gray matter in spinal cord sections remained similar to controls, in spite of reduced cross-sectional area [17]. These results suggest that atrophy of MS spinal cords affects both gray and white matter equally. Neuronal degeneration caused by gray matter lesions might result in gray matter atrophy [36, 39, 40]. In addition, axonal transection in white matter might cause retrograde degeneration of gray matter neurons [8].

N-acetyl Aspartate as a Marker for Axonal Injury in MS

The role of axonal injury in MS suggests that non-invasive monitoring could be useful for the study of disease progression as well as evaluation of ongoing therapy in these patients. Although a correlation between axon loss and hypointensity in T1-weighted images has been suggested in MS [7, 41], MRI generally lacks pathological specificity, as many factors can influence image contrast [5, 42]. Measurements of *N*-acetyl aspartate (NAA) levels by proton MRS is therefore a valuable tool for non-invasive in vivo monitoring of disease progression in general and axonal pathology in particular.

NAA is the second most-abundant amino acid in the adult CNS after glutamate, and is localized primarily in neurons and neuronal processes [43-45]. After synthesis in mitochondria from L-apartate and acetyl-CoA, NAA is transported to the cytoplasm where it is present in high concentrations [46, 47]. The function of NAA is unknown, although participation in protein synthesis, osmotic regulation, myelination, and metabolism of neurotransmitters such as aspartate and *N*-acetyl-glutamate has been suggested [43, 48-50]. Decreased levels of NAA, as measured by MRS, have been demonstrated in a number of neurodegenerative disorders, including MS [5, 51, 52]. In acute stages of MS, reduced NAA is partly reversible, restricted to lesion area, and correlates with reversible functional impairment [2, 15, 53, 54]. In chronic stages of MS, reduced NAA is also detected in normal-appearing white matter, suggesting axonal damage or Wallerian degeneration outside MS lesions [5, 55, 56]. In addition, NAA levels correlate with disability over time in patients with MS [2, 5, 56]. Recently, Lee et al. [57] investigated the relationship between tract-specific NAA reductions and motor impairment in MS patients by measuring NAA levels and central motor conduction times in normal-appearing capsula interna bilaterally. The data show side-to-side correlations between levels of NAA, conduction times, and motor impairment, indicating that MRS measured axonal pathology in non-lesion white matter is a precise determinant of disease progression in MS [57]. In SPMS spinal cords, average NAA levels were significantly decreased by 53% and 55% at cervical and lumbar levels, respectively, as determined by high-performance liquid chromatography (HPLC) [17]. Since these patients were severely disabled (EDSS $\geq$ 7.5), the data indicate that reduced NAA levels in chronic MS can reflect irreversible functional impairment.

Reduced NAA levels in MS could reflect reversible neuronal/axonal damage due to inflammatory demyelination, altered neuronal/axonal metabolism related to activity, axonal atrophy, or axonal loss [2, 5, 15, 58]. To differentiate these mechanisms, spinal cord NAA, measured by postmortem HPLC, was correlated with axonal loss, as determined by immunohistochemistry in MS lesions, MS non-lesions, and control white matter (Fig. 4A-F) [17]. Both total axonal volume and tissue concentration of NAA was significantly reduced in the chronic inactive lesions. The average decrease in axonal density of 62% in these lesions demonstrates that reduced NAA levels correlate with substantial axonal loss. These data support axonal loss as a major cause of reduced NAA levels in chronic stages of MS. In order to investigate whether axonal loss is the only contributor to decreased levels of NAA in chronic MS spinal cords, NAA per axonal volume was calculated (Fig. 4G) [17]. Compared with myelinated axons in control white matter, average NAA per axonal volume was reduced in myelinated axons in MS non-lesion white matter by 30% ($p=0.05$), and in demyelinated axons in MS lesions by 42% ($p=0.01$). These data indicate that NAA metabolism is related to neuronal activity in a tract. Since these MS patients were non-ambulatory, the 30% reduction of NAA in normal-appearing myelinated axons supports reduced NAA in the absence of demyelination in axons functionally impaired due to paralysis. Acute deafferentation in the CNS causes trans-synaptic decreases of NAA levels without ultrastructural abnormalities, indicating that denervation and/or impaired function reduces neuronal NAA [59]. Hence, denervation of a neuron due to damage of afferent axons, for example in remote lesions, may cause altered NAA levels. Demyelinated axons

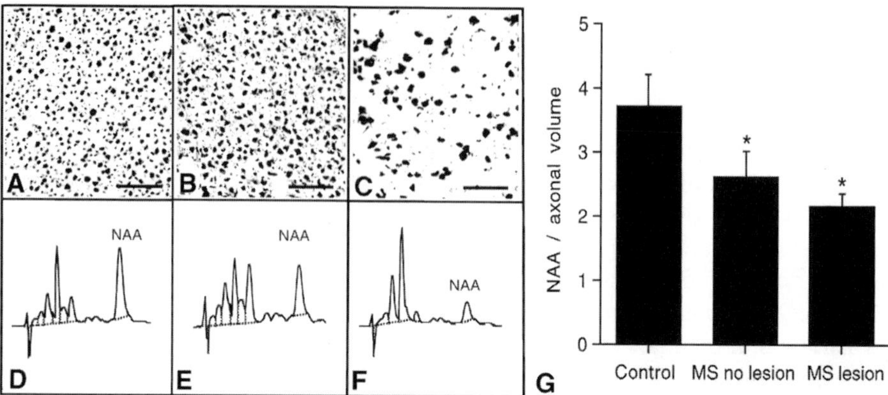

Fig. 4. Correlation between loss of axons and levels of *N*-acetyl aspartate (NAA) in MS spinal cord white matter. Axonal volume and density was determined in neurofilament-stained cryostat sections and NAA levels were determined by high-performance liquid chromatography (HPLC) in adjacent sections. *Top panel,* representative micrographs showing axons in control white matter (**A**), MS white matter without lesion (**B**), and in an MS lesion (**C**). Scale bars = 40 μm. *Lower panel,* HPLC chromatograms (**D, E, F**) from tissue sections adjacent to those immunostained in (**A**), (**B**) and (**C**), respectively. Levels of NAA per axonal volume in myelinated and demyelinated axons in control and MS samples (**G**). Average NAA per axonal volume was significantly reduced in MS non-lesion white matter samples (30%, *p*=0.05) and in samples from chronic MS lesions (42%, *p*=0.01). From [17]

contained 42% less NAA than myelinated axons in control spinal cords. Demyelination and remyelination influence axonal neurofilament phoshporylation dynamically by regulating kinase and phosphatase activity locally [60]. It is possible that local axonal enzymes involved in NAA metabolism are affected by the state of myelination in a similar manner. Finally, since NAA is synthesized in mitochondria [46, 47], changes in NAA could reflect mitochondrial dysfunction [61]. For example, local inflammation may indirectly influence mitochondrial function. In acute EAE, an animal model of MS characterized by inflammation and demyelination, mitochondrial dysfunction and reduced NAA has been reported in the absence of neuronal loss [61-63].

Neurological Disability and Axonal Pathology

The data discussed in this review suggest that axonal injury begins at the onset of MS, and that cumulative axonal loss provides the pathological substrate for permanent disability in affected patients. However, since the CNS has a remarkable ability to compensate for neuronal loss, axonal injury and degeneration may remain subclinical for many years [1, 8, 64]. Interestingly, an average axonal loss of 64% was observed in MS lesions from individuals without clinical impairment

[65]. The lack of neurological symptoms was suggested to reflect lesion site, neuronal redundancy, moderate total axon loss, and remyelination.

Episodes of reversible clinical symptoms during RRMS are primarily associated with acute inflammatory lesions in articulate parts of the CNS. It is believed that four mechanisms contribute to clinical remission: resolution of the inflammation, redistribution of axolemmal sodium channels, remyelination, and adaptive cortical changes [1]. A recent combined functional MRI and MRS study of RRMS patients without overt permanent functional disability demonstrated a fivefold increase in sensorimotor cortex activation after simple hand movements when compared with control individuals [66]. These results suggest that compensatory cortical changes, possibly involving reorganization of functional pathways, may contribute to maintained motor function after axonal damage during early MS.

Since demyelinated axons can regain their ability to conduct impulses after axolemmal remodeling [67, 68], it is unlikely that demyelination is the only cause of chronic disability in MS [5, 6, 8]. The magnitude of axonal loss in chronic spinal cord lesions from severely disabled patients, and the reduction of NAA levels in MS tissue with time, support the hypothesis that the transition from RRMS to SPMS occurs when a threshold of neuronal or axonal loss is reached [1, 8, 17, 18, 69, 70]. The time at which a patient develops permanent disability, SPMS, varies between individuals, and probably reflects a number of factors, such as location of lesions, disease activity, medication, and various aspects of genetic susceptibility. An epidemiological study by Confavreaux et al. [71] showed that although the time from disease onset to EDSS score 4 varied between 1 and 33 years, the time course from EDSS score 4 to EDSS score 7 was similar among the 1,844 MS patients included in the study. These data support the hypothesis that many MS patients eventually enter a final common pathway of progressive CNS degeneration once a clinical threshold is reached. Hence, the extent of inflammatory demyelination may influence the time course to EDSS score 4. However, since the subsequent progression to EDSS score 7 continued in the absence of inflammatory lesions, it is possible that preprogrammed neurodegeneration is a factor behind the functional decline experienced by most SPMS patients [1, 23].

The concept of MS as an inflammatory neurodegenerative disease has important implications regarding treatment strategies. Since lesions can outnumber clinical relapses by as much as 10:1 [72], continuous inflammation may cause considerable tissue damage in the absence of obvious clinical manifestations. Anti-inflammatory and immunomodulatory treatment might therefore also provide indirect neuroprotection. A number of drugs with a documented effect during RRMS are now available, for example interferon β and glatiramer acetate [23, 73]. Disease-modifying therapy should be used early and continuously in order to prevent and delay accumulating axonal degeneration, and thereby prevent and delay development of permanent functional disability [64]. SPMS is characterized by decreasing response to anti-inflammatory treatment, and satisfactory therapies for progressive MS are currently lacking. Since chronic demyelinated axons might undergo degeneration due to lack of trophic support provided by myelin, promotion of remyelination by endogenous oligodendrocytes, or transplantation of myelinating cells, could be feasible future treatment strategies for chronic stages of MS. The role of cumulative axonal degeneration in the development of permanent disability in MS also suggests that neuroprotective therapies should be added to the anti-inflammatory and immunomodulatory treatments presently used for MS patients. The development of neuroprotective drugs that apply to MS should therefore be a priority for MS research.

Acknowledgments. This work was supported by NIH grants NS35058, NS38667 and by a pilot study grant (B.D.T.) and a postdoctoral fellowship (C.B.) from the National Multiple Sclerosis Society. The authors thank Dr. Grahame Kidd for assistance with the illustrations.

References

1. Bjartmar C, Trapp BD (2001) Axonal and neuronal degeneration in multiple sclerosis: mechanisms and functional consequences. Curr Opin Neurol 14:271-278
2. Arnold DL et al (1994) Use of proton magnetic resonance spectroscopy for monitoring disease progression in multiple sclerosis. Ann Neurol 36:76-82
3. De Stefano N et al (1998) Axonal damage correlates with disability in patients with relapsing-remitting multiple sclerosis. Results of a longitudinal magnetic resonance spectroscopy study. Brain 121:1469-1477
4. Trapp BD et al (1998) Axonal transection in the lesions of multiple sclerosis. N Engl J Med 338:278-285
5. Matthews PM et al (1998) Putting magnetic resonance spectroscopy studies in context: axonal damage and disability in multiple sclerosis. Semin Neurol 18:327-336
6. Bjartmar C, Yin X, Trapp BD (1999) Axonal pathology in myelin disorders. J Neurocytol 28:383-395
7. van Waesberghe JHTM et al (1999) Axonal loss in multiple sclerosis lesions: magnetic resonance imaging insights into substrates of disability. Ann Neurol 46:747-754
8. Trapp BD, Ransohoff RM, Fisher E, Rudick RA (1999) Neurodegeneration in multiple sclerosis: relationship to neurological disability. Neuroscientist 5:48-57
9. Ferguson B, Matyszak MK, Esiri MM, Perry VH (1997) Axonal damage in acute multiple sclerosis lesions. Brain 120:393-399
10. Kornek B, Lassman H (1999) Axonal pathology in multiple sclerosis. A historical note. Brain Pathol 9:651-656
11. Charcot M (1868) Histologie de le sclerose en plaques. Gazette Hopitaux 141:554-558
12. Davie CA et al (1995) Persistent functional deficit in multiple sclerosis and autosomal dominant cerebellar ataxia is associated with axon loss. Brain 118:1583-1592
13. Losseff NA et al (1996) Spinal cord atrophy and disability in multiple sclerosis. A new reproducible and sensitive MRI method with potential to monitor disease progression. Brain 119:701-708
14. Losseff NA et al (1996) Progressive cerebral atrophy in multiple sclerosis. A serial MRI study. Brain 119:2009-2019
15. Narayana PA, Doyle TJ, Dejian L, Wolinsky JS (1998) Serial proton magnetic resonance spectroscopic imaging, contrast-enhanced magnetic resonance imaging, and quantitative lesion volumetry in multiple sclerosis. Ann Neurol 43:56-71

16. Scherer S (1999) Axonal pathology in demyelinating diseases. Ann Neurol 45:6-7
17. Bjartmar C et al (2000) Neurological disability correlates with spinal cord axonal loss and reduced *N*-acetyl-aspartate in chronic multiple sclerosis patients. Ann Neurol 48:893-901
18. Lovas G et al (2000) Axonal changes in chronic demyelinated cervical spinal cord plaques. Brain 123:308-317
19. Koo EH et al (1990) Precursor of amyloid protein in Alzheimer disease undergoes fast anterograde axonal transport. Proc Nat Acad Sci USA 87:1561-1565
20. Hohlfeld R (1997) Biotechnological agents for the immunotherapy of multiple sclerosis. Principles, problems and perspectives. Brain 120:865-916
21. Bell JI, Lathrop GM (1996) Multiple loci for multiple sclerosis. Nature Genet 13:377-378
22. Ebers GC, Dyment DA (1998) Genetics of multiple sclerosis. Semin Neurol 18:295-299
23. Noseworthy JH, Luccinetti C, Rodriquez M, Weinshenker BG (2000) Multiple sclerosis. N Engl J Med 343:938-952
24. Rivera-Quinones C et al (1998) Absence of neurological deficits following extensive demyelination in a class I-deficient murine model of multiple sclerosis. Nat Med 4:187-193
25. Njenga MK et al (1999) Absence of spontaneous central nervous system remyelination in class II-deficient mice infected with Theiler´s virus. J Neuropathol Exp Neurol 58:78-91
26. Giese KP et al (1992) Mouse P0 gene disruption leads to hypomyelination, abnormal expression of recognition molecules, and degeneration of myelin and axons. Cell 71:565-576
27. Anzini P et al (1997) Structural abnormalities and deficient maintenance of peripheral nerve myelin in mice lacking the gap junction protein connexin 32. J Neurosci 17:4545-4551
28. Yin X et al (1998) Myelin-associated glycoprotein is a myelin signal that modulates the caliber of myelinated axons. J Neurosci 18:1953-1962
29. Griffiths I et al (1998) Axonal swellings and degeneration in mice lacking the major proteolipid of myelin. Science 280:1610-1613
30. Sahenk Z, Chen L, Mendell JR (1999) Effects of PMP22 duplication and deletions on the axonal cytoskeleton. Ann Neurol 45:16-24
31. Ganter P, Prince C, Esiri MM (1999) Spinal cord axonal loss in multiple sclerosis: a post-mortem study. Neuropathol Appl Neurobiol 25:459-467
32. Evangelou N et al (2000) Quantitative pathological evidence for axonal loss in normal appearing white matter in multiple sclerosis. Ann Neurol 47:391-395
33. Stevenson VL, Miller DH (1999) Magnetic resonance imaging in the monitoring of disease progression in multiple sclerosis. Multiple Sclerosis 5:268-272
34. Kidd D et al (1993) Spinal cord MRI using multi-array coils and fast spin echo. II. Findings in multiple sclerosis. Neurology 43:2632-2637
35. Filippi M et al (1997) A longitudinal magnetic resonance imaging study of the cervical cord in multiple sclerosis. J Neuroimaging 7:78-80
36. Brownell B, Hughes JT (1962) The distribution of plaques in the cerebrum in multiple sclerosis. J Neurol Neurosurg Psychiatry 25:315-320
37. Simon JH et al (1999) A longitudinal study of brain atrophy in relapsing multiple sclerosis. Neurology 53:139-148
38. Rudick RA et al (1999) Use of the brain parenchymal fraction to measure whole brain atrophy in relapsing-remitting MS. Multiple Sclerosis Collaborative Research Group. Neurology 53:1698-1704
39. Lumsden CE (1970) The neuropathology of multiple sclerosis. In: Vinken PJ, Bruyn GW (eds) Handbook of clinical neurology, vol 9. North-Holland, Amsterdam, pp 217-309

40. Kidd D et al (1999) Cortical lesions in multiple sclerosis. Brain 122:17-26
41. van Walderveen MAA et al (1998) Histopathologic correlate of hypointense lesions on T1-weighted spin-echo MRI in multiple sclerosis. Neurology 50:1282-1288
42. Brück W et al (1997) Inflammatory central nervous system demyelination: correlation of magnetic resonance imaging findings with lesion pathology. Ann Neurol 42:783-793
43. Baslow MH (2000) Functions of N-acetyl-L-aspartate and *N*-acetyl-L-aspartylglutamate in the vertebrate brain: role in glial cell-specific signaling. J Neurochem 75:453-459
44. Moffett JR, Namboodiri MAA, Cangro CB, Neale JH (1991) Immunohistochemical localization of *N*-acetylaspartate in rat brain. Neuroreport 2:131-134
45. Simmons ML, Frondoza CG, Coyle JT (1991) Immunocytochemical localization of *N*-acetyl-aspartate with monoclonal antibodies. Neuroscience 45:37-45
46. Patel TB, Clark JB (1979) Synthesis of *N*-acetyl-L-aspartate by rat brain mitochondria and involvement in mitochondrial/cytosolic carbon transport. Biochem J 184:539-546
47. Truckenmiller ME, Namboodiri MAA, Brownstein MJ, Neale JH (1985) *N*-acetylation of L-aspartate in the nervous system: differential distribution of a specific enzyme. J Neurochem 45:1658-1662
48. Clarke DD et al (1975) A relationship of *N*-acetylaspartate biosynthesis to neuronal protein synthesis. J Neurochem 24:479-485
49. Cangro CB et al (1987) Immunohistochemistry and biosynthesis of *N*-acetylaspartylglutamate in spinal sensory ganglia. J Neurochem 49:1579-1588
50. Lee JH, Arcinue E, Ross BD (1994) Brief report: organic osmolytes in the brain of an infant with hypernatremia. N Engl J Med 331:439-442
51. Graham GD et al (1992) Proton magnetic resonance spectroscopy of cerebral lactate and other metabolites in stroke patients. Stroke 23:333-340
52. Pioro E, Antel JP, Cashman NR, Arnold DL (1994) Detection of cortical neuron loss in motor neuron disease by proton magnetic resonance spectroscopic imaging in vivo. Neurology 44:1933-1938
53. Davie CA et al (1994) Serial proton magnetic resonance spectroscopy in acute multiple sclerosis lesions. Brain 117:49-58
54. Matthews PM et al (1996) Assessment of lesion pathology in multiple sclerosis using quantitative MRI morphometry and magnetic resonance spectroscopy. Brain 119:715-722
55. Narayanan S et al (1997) Imaging of axonal damage in multiple sclerosis: spatial distribution of magnetic resonance imaging lesions. Ann Neurol 41:385-391
56. Fu L et al (1998) Imaging axonal damage of normal-appearing white matter in multiple sclerosis. Brain 121:103-113
57. Lee MA et al (2000) Axonal injury or loss in the internal capsule and motor impairment in multiple sclerosis. Arch Neurol 57:65-70
58. De Stefano N, Matthews PM, Arnold DL (1995) Reversible decreases in *N*-acetylaspartate after acute brain injury. Magn Reson Med 34:721-727
59. Rango M et al (1995) Central nervous system trans-synaptic effects of acute axonal injury: a ^{1}H magnetic resonance spectroscopy study. Magn Reson Med 33:595-600
60. de Waegh SM, Lee VM-Y, Brady ST (1992) Local modulation of neurofilament phosphorylation, axonal caliber, and slow axonal transport by myelinating Schwann cells. Cell 68:451-463
61. Clark JB (1998) *N*-Acetyl aspartate: a marker for neuronal loss or mitochondrial dysfunction. Dev Neurosci 20:271-276
62. Saragea M et al (1965) Biochemical changes occurring in animals with experimental allergic encephalomyelitis. Med Pharmacol Exp 13:74-80
63. Brenner RE et al (1993) The proton NMR spectrum in acute EAE: the significance of the change in the Cho:Cr ratio. Magn Reson Med 29:737-745

64. Rudick RA, Goodman A, Herndon RM, Panitch HS (1999) Selecting relapsing remitting multiple sclerosis patients for treatment: the case for early treatment. J Neuroimmunol 98:22-28
65. Mews I et al (1998) Oligodendrocyte and axon pathology in clinically silent multiple sclerosis lesions. Multiple Sclerosis 4:55-62
66. Reddy H et al (2000) Evidence for adaptive functional changes in the cerebral cortex with axonal injury from multiple sclerosis. Brain 123:2314-2320
67. Foster RE, Whalen CC, Waxman SG (1980) Reorganization of the axon membrane in demyelinated peripheral nerve fibers: morphological evidence. Science 210:661-663
68. Felts PA, Baker TA, Smith KJ (1997) Conduction in segmentally demyelinated mammalian central axons. J Neurosci 17:7267-7277
69. Waxman SG (1998) Demyelinating diseases – new pathological insights, new therapeutic targets. N Engl J Med 338:223-225
70. Gonen O et al (2000) Total brain N-acetylaspartate. A new measure of disease load in MS. Neurology 54:15-19
71. Confavreux C, Vukusic S, Moreau T, Adeleine P (2000) Relapses and progression of disability in multiple sclerosis. N Engl J Med 343:1430-1438
72. McFarland HF et al (1992) Using gadolinium-enhanced magnetic resonance imaging lesions to monitor disease activity in multiple sclerosis. Ann Neurol 32:758-766
73. Rudick RA et al (1997) Management of multiple sclerosis. N Engl J Med 337:1604-1611
74. Trapp BD, Ransohoff R, Rudick R (1999) Axonal pathology in multiple sclerosis: relationship to neurologic disability. Curr Opin Neurol 12:295-302

Chapter 6

Autoimmune Inflammation and Multiple Sclerosis

I.R. COHEN

Inflammation and Multiple Sclerosis

The term inflammation was first used as a gross description of the redness of the skin observed at sites of injury. Later it was discovered that the redness was the natural result of blood vessel physiology. Now we know that the blood vessels are only one of the many factors involved in inflammation, a process in which immune cells of various types and their molecular products interact with signal molecules produced by the injured tissue.

There are different ways to view the roles of inflammation, depending much on the aspect of your view. Lord Florey quotes Ebert who proposed that "inflammation is a process that begins following a sublethal injury to tissue and ends with complete healing" [1]. Florey invoked Ebert to stress the idea that "inflammation is a process and not a state. The inflamed area undergoes continuous change." Inflammation, in Florey's view, is a process that is initiated by injury and aims at healing. What then is the role of inflammation in multiple sclerosis (MS), particularly the inflammation caused by autoimmunity?

Healing is not the traditional role assigned to inflammation in MS. On the contrary, inflammation is seen as the cause of MS; autoimmunity to myelin triggers aberrant inflammation, and this inflammation injures the white matter of the central nervous system (CNS) producing MS. Inflammation, even physiological inflammation, triggers the death of cells and the remodeling of tissue [2]. Cell death and scar formation is decidedly not good for the CNS; indeed, immune privilege may have evolved to isolate the CNS from inflammation of any kind [3]. Inflammation in the CNS, even if bent on healing, may complicate rather than cure disease. Is inflammation then the pathogenic culprit in MS, or could it be a physiological healer of MS?

We are now beginning to appreciate the molecular complexity of inflammation and its spectrum of manifestations; inflammation activates genes and makes some cells die, some cells move, and some cells proliferate and differentiate [2]. Inflammation remodels connective tissue and triggers angiogenesis and vascular adjustment. Inflammation can be critical in inducing tissue regeneration; activated macrophages can even trigger regeneration of the injured CNS [4]. Inflammation, then, is not of one type; inflammation is a manifold agent for body maintenance. If this is really the case, we ought to consider the possibility that some of the inflammatory manifestations of MS are reparative, and not all bad. The problem, of course, is to sort out the good from the bad. In either case, blind immunosuppression is likely to disable the good along with the bad.

Autoimmunity and MS

Autoimmunity refers to a process in which the antigen receptors of lymphocytes are capable of recognizing antigens in the individual's healthy tissues [2]. Because autoimmunity requires antigen receptors, the phenomenon of autoimmunity is a property of the adaptive arm of the immune system. Inflammation, however, is the outcome of the activation of both the innate and adaptive arms of the immune system; the cytokines and other molecules that orchestrate inflammation are produced both by the adaptive T cells and B cells and by the innate leukocytes [5]. The role of autoimmunity in MS is thus related to the role of inflammation in MS.

Autoimmunity used to be equated with disease; it was inconceivable that healthy individuals might harbor autoimmune lymphocytes in their immune systems [6]. The immune system was viewed as a defense system only; a system that attacked whatever molecules it might be able to recognize. Such a system could only live in peace with the body if the system were purged of antigen receptors capable of self-recognition. Autoimmune disease, therefore, was imagined to erupt whenever an autoimmune lymphocyte accidentally appeared. Autoimmunity could never be up to any good.

This classic concept of autoimmunity is logical, but it does not comply with the facts; autoimmune B cells are common in every body housing an adaptive immune system [7, 8], yet most bodies show no evidence of autoimmune disease. Moreover, the activation of autoimmune T cells can contribute to maintenance of the body. My colleagues and I have shown that lines and clones of T cells reactive to myelin can cause the MS-like disease – experimental autoimmune encephalomelitis [9]. However, these same T cells were found to mediate neuroprotection when applied to the models of CNS white matter injury developed by Schwartz and colleagues [10-12]. Inflammatory processes involving autoimmune T cells, like those mediated by innate leukocytes [4], can promote healing [10, 11]. Moreover, autoimmune T cells that recognize myelin seem to be activated as a matter of course in CNS injury [13]. Thus we return to the questions of cause and effect; is the activation of autoimmunity observed in MS a result of the disease, or is activated autoimmunity the cause of disease?

Causality and MS

The problem with the cause-and-effect questions is that neither inflammation nor autoimmunity are intrinsically good or bad; the outcomes of inflammation and of autoimmunity depend on the circumstances. Sometimes these processes are beneficial and sometimes they are detrimental. So we cannot reduce MS to CNS white matter autoimmune inflammation. MS emerges from inappropriate interactions, not from faulty parts [2]. MS is a basket of reaction patterns; similar reaction patterns may be triggered off by different factors, such as viral infections, traumatic injury, stress, and so forth. Autoimmunity to myelin is built into the normal immune system physiologically; myelin autoimmunity is a part of the immunological homunculus [8, 14, 15]. The disease erupts when the autoimmune process is unleashed, by whatever insult, and when the process gets stuck in a mode of recurrent or chronic activation.

Treatment for MS

MS is a complex disease because both the brain and the immune system are complex systems. Indeed, inflammation and autoimmunity are complex manifestations of the immune system. So how are we to deal with MS? Ideally, it is usually more efficient and less costly in side-effects to go with nature, than against nature. If autoimmune inflammation has the capacity to heal, as well as harm, it might be useful to enlist the immune system itself to regulate the type, timing, site, and strength of inflammation that takes place in the patient. β-interferon is a modulator of immune inflammation and Copaxone also exerts multiple effects on the autoimmune response. T-cell vaccination was thought to work primarily by inducing anti-idiotypic regulation, but now we are discovering that T-cell vaccination actually affects the nature of the cytokines generated by the autoimmune response [16, 17 18, 19]. T-cell vaccination, thus, influences the nature of autoimmune inflammation.

Modulation of autoimmune inflammation, by whatever means, is likely to be more successful if it is instituted as early as possible in the course of the disease, before detrimental feed-back loops become entrenched. Moreover, we need convenient methods to monitor the state of the immune system and its response to treatment. Each patient, because of individual genetics and individual immune history, is likely to need different forms of treatment, doses, and dose scheduling to obtain an optimal therapeutic effect. The new bioinformatics might be deployed to stage the immune system and its response to therapy in MS and in other autoimmune diseases [2].

Acknowledgements. I am the incumbent of the Mauerberger Chair of Immunology and the Director of the Robert Koch-Minerva Centre for Research of Autoimmune Diseases. I thank Ms. Danielle Sabah-Israel for her help in preparing this manuscript.

References

1. Florey HW (1970) General pathology, 4th ed Lloyd-Luke, London, pp 22-39
2. Cohen IR (2000) Tending Adam's garden: evolving the cognative immune self. Academic Press, London

3. Schwartz M, Moalem G, Leibowitz-Amit, Cohen IR (1999) Innate and adaptive immune responses can be beneficial for CNS repair. Trends Neurosci 22:295-299
4. Schwartz M, Lazarov-Speigler O (1998) The role of immune system in central nervous system recovery: an evolutionary perspective. Curr Top Neurochem 1:123-132
5. Cohen IR (2000) Discrimination and dialogue in the immune system. Semin Immunol 12:215-219
6. Burnel M (1959) Self and not self. Cambridge University Press, Cambridge
7. Avarameas S (1991) Natural autoantibodies from "Horro Autotoxicus" to "Gnothi Seauton". Immunol Today 12:154-159
8. Cohen IR (1992) The cognitive paradigm and the immunological homunculus. Immunol Today 13:490-494
9. Ben-Nun A, Wekerle H, Cohen IR (1981) The rapid isolation of clonable antigen-specific T lymphocyte lines capable of mediating autoimmune encephalomyelitis. Eur J Immunol 11:195-199
10. Moalem G et al (1999) Autoimmune T cells protect neurons from secondary degeneration after central nervous system axotomy. Nat Med 5:49-55
11. Hauben E et al (2000) Autoimmune T cells as potential neuroprotective therapy for spinal cord injury. Lancet 355:286-287
12. Schwartz M, Cohen IR (2000) Autoimmunity can benefit self-maintenance. Immunol Today 21:265-268
13. Yoles E et al (2001) Protective autoimmunity is a physiological response to CNS trauma. J Neurosci 21:3740-3748
14. Cohen IR, Young DB (1991) Autoimmunity, microbial immunity and the immunological homunculus. Immunol Today 12:105-110
15. Cohen IR (1992) The cognitive principle challenges clonal selection. Immunol Today 13:441-444
16. Elias D, Tikochinski Y, Frankel G, Cohen IR (1999) Regulation of NOD mouse autoimmune diabetes by T cells that recognize a TCR CDR3 peptide. Int Immunol 11:957-966
17. Waisman A et al (1996) Suppressive vaccination with DNA encoding a variable region gene of the T-cell receptor prevents autoimmune encephalomyelitis and activates Th2 immunity. Nat Med 2:899-905
18. Zang YC, Hong J, Tejada-Simon MV, Li S, Rivera VM, Killian JM, Zhang JZ (2000) Th2 immune regulation induced by T cell vaccination in patients with multiple sclerosis. Eur J Immunol 30:908-913
19. Zang YC, Hong J, Rivera VM, Killian J, Zhang JZ (2000) Preferential recognition of TCR hypervariable regions by human anti-idiotipic T cells induced by T cell vaccination. J Immunol 164:4011-4017

Chapter 7

Early Treatment of Progression in Multiple Sclerosis

R.E. GONSETTE

Introduction

Progression is a clinical concept linked to a gradual, irreversible increase in disability that correlates with the transition from the relapsing-remitting (RR) to the progressive stages. It is becoming increasingly clear that progressive multiple sclerosis (MS) is associated with axonal loss and that axonal damage occurs early during RRMS. Disease progression thus develops well in advance of clinical progression and remains subclinical because, due to compensatory mechanisms, impairment does not interfere with daily living activities at that stage.

These new emerging concepts about MS pathogenesis imply that therapeutic approaches to delay progression should be started as soon as possible after MS onset. This paper will concern potential intervention during the early stages of MS, either to delay the transition from the RR phase to the progressive phase or to block frequent severe relapses leading to the early development of disability.

Prevention of Early Progression Due to Inflammatory and Oxidative Mechanisms

Pathomechanisms of Early Lesions

Immune-mediated mechanisms leading to early myelin destruction are well known [1]: striping by macrophages, vesicular disruption mediated by antibody dependent cytotoxicity, attachment of microglia to myelin internodes, reaction with opsonized myelin through Fc and complement receptors, as well as production of various myelinolytic factors [cytokines, reactive nitrogen species (RNS), reactive oxygen species (ROS), and other free radicals].

The mechanisms mediating axonal damage are less clear [2]. There is no evidence so far that axons can be directly destroyed by the immune system, like in acute motor axonal neuropathy. Early axonal damage seems the result of a two-step mechanism: first, axonal demyelination caused by immune-mediated inflammation; second, destruction of demyelinated axons by toxic mediators released by macrophages and activated microglia in the inflammatory environment. It appears that, in addition to proteolytic enzymes, lesions of demyelinated axons result for the most part from non-specific oxidative products [3] and that this process may continue even after inflammatory reactions have subsided. It has been demonstrated that axonal conduction can be blocked reversibly by nitric oxide (NO•) [4], specifically in axons displaying evidence of demyelination, whereas normal axons usually remain unaffected. Moreover, after exposure to higher concentrations, this blocking effect becomes persistent, even if NO• is removed [5].

During the early stage of the disease, oligodendrocytes do not seem the primary target of the inflammatory response, except in acute cases. However, repeated destruction of oligodendrocytes even by low levels of oxidative toxicity [6-8] will lead progressively to the deletion not only of oligodendrocytes but also of mature progenitor cells.

Mickel [9] suggested in 1975 that myelin degradation might be the result of lipid peroxidation mediated by lipid peroxides arising from the gastrointestinal tract, but the role of these non-specific toxic factors in MS pathology was underestimated until recently. There is converging evidence today that demyelination and axonal loss involve both immune-mediated inflammatory and oxidative mechanisms, and that therapeutic efforts should target both of them.

Oxidative Mechanisms Possibly Involved in MS

Free hydroxyl radical (OH•) is the ROS of primary concern. The mean substrate for OH• production is hydrogen peroxide (H_2O_2). In addition to NO• and superoxide (O_2^-), activation of macrophages produces H_2O_2. Both O_2 and NO• release iron from ferritin [10] (an iron storage protein present in various cell types, including macrophages), which in turn catalyzes the decay of H_2O_2 to OH• [11]. It is noteworthy that iron is also abundant in myelin and that myelin degradation releases H_2O_2, the required substrate for OH• formation [12]. However, mammalian cells are equipped with high concentrations of antioxidant enzymes [particularly superoxide dismutase (SOD)] capable of quenching OH• effectively [11], and the role of OH• in MS pathology appears therefore limited.

RNS seem to play a major role in toxic oxidative mechanisms. Under physiological conditions, the free radical NO• is produced by the interaction of constitutive nitric oxide synthase (cNOS) with L-arginine and mediates a variety of normal biological functions, such as immunoregulation of inflammatory reactions, downregulation of tumor necrosis factor-α (TNF-α) production, MHC II expression on macrophages, induction of apoptosis in specific CD4 cells, and inhibition of antigen presentation as well as leukocyte adhesion and migration [13-16]. During inflammatory reactions, however, exposure of macrophages to interferon-γ (IFN-γ) and TNF-α leads to the activation of the inducible form of NOS (iNOS) [17] and, subsequently, to the production in close vicinity and for extended periods of high levels of NO• and superoxide (O_2^-). These two molecules interact at a rate three times faster than the rate at which SOD scavenges O_2^- to form peroxynitrite ($ONOO^-$) in large amounts, a very potent oxidant. The role of NO• in MS is thus complex, and it is very likely that its derivatives, particularly ONOO⁻, are definitely more toxic than NO• itself.

What makes ONOO⁻ particularly toxic is its remarkable stability as an anion at alkaline pH, allowing a greater opportunity to diffuse through a cell to find a target [16]. At acid pH, peroxynitrite, which is not a free radical, is protonated to form peroxinitrous acid and is catalyzed by transition metals to generate OH• and nitronium anion (NO_2^+) that produces nitrophenols and nitrotyrosine (NT). Although ONOO⁻ may also decay into OH•, its own oxidizing effects appear more damaging because they occur much faster than OH• formation. As a result, the RNS pathway is likely the most important for free radical toxicity in MS and ONOO⁻ is definitely the most-toxic molecule.

Oxidative Toxicity in MS

Since the first publication [9], several investigations have been performed to elucidate the role of oxidative mechanisms in MS and in its animal model, experimental allergic encephalomyelitis (EAE). An increased oxidative metabolism in serum or in blood cells from MS patients was first reported [18, 19]. It was suggested that monocytes, stimulated by IFN-γ, had a crucial role [20], and this was confirmed later [12].

An increased production of H_2O_2 and O_2^- by stimulated monocytes from MS patients was demonstrated [21], and elevated serum lipid peroxidation products were found in rapidly progressive MS [22]. This was not observed in a further study that reported an enhanced generation of O_2^- during relapses [23]. More recently, one paper excepted [24], several publications demonstrated significantly elevated serum levels of NO_2 and NO_3 in MS compared with other neurological diseases [25]. Serial determinations revealed that this elevation correlates with a relapsing course [26, 27].

Several other converging observations are also strongly suggestive of an increased oxidative metabolism in MS patients: raised NT serum levels [28], immune response of MS patients to nitroso-amino acid conjugates [29], consumption of non-enzymatic antioxidants during relapses [30], and a higher concentration of the reduced form of sulfydryl groups of glutathione [31].

Increased lipid peroxidation products in the cerebrospinal fluid (CSF) of MS patients was reported in 1985 [32], but the demonstration of a highly significant increase of NO_2 and/or NO_3 content in CSF provided for the first evidence of abnormal NO• production in the central nervous system (CNS) of MS patients [26, 33]. Those levels are markedly elevated during exacerbations and are effectively suppressed with intravenous methylprednisolone [34]. Recent studies report that NO_2 but not NO_3 is elevated in MS [35], whereas increased CSF levels of these two molecules are questioned in some papers [36, 37]. Isoprostane, a marker of oxidative stress in vivo, is definitely higher in MS patients and lowered by steroid treatment [38].

It was first suggested in pathological studies [39] that the increase in uric acid (which is considered as a marker for free radical activity) concomitant with a decrease in glutathione (the main water-soluble antioxidant) in plaques compared with surrounding white matter reflected abnormal oxidative mechanisms in MS patients.

The first direct demonstration of NOS in regions of MS brains undergoing active demyelination was in 1994 [14, 40] with immunocytochemical techniques localizing NADPH-diaphorase activity. NOS was colocalized with astrocyte staining. However, NADPH does not distinguish between cNOS and iNOS. Further studies with specific anti-iNOS and anti-cNOS antibodies [41, 42] confirmed an increased production of iNOS in acute but not in chronic plaques. Constitutive NOS was colocalized with astrocyte and endothelial cell staining, whereas iNOS was colocalized with microglia and macrophages.

Nitrotyrosine, a product of the nitration of thyrosine by $ONOO^-$, is used as a specific and stable marker of this oxidant and confirms the generation of $ONOO^-$ in actively demyelinating lesions [43]. Other techniques have also demonstrated oxidative damage in MS brains: increased DNA oxidation [44] and infrared spectroscopy showing lipid and protein oxidation in active lesion sites [45]. Importantly, all studies show that the presence of RNS and/or ROS is closely associated with acute inflammatory lesions, and is rarely observed in chronic inactive plaques [41-43, 46].

Experimental Prevention of Oxidative Toxicity

Experiments in EAE animal models have been conducted to elucidate the mechanisms of oxidative toxicity and to evaluate the effects of several compounds potentially useful for reducing myelin and axonal damage in MS patients. It was demonstrated in acute EAE that NO• plays a role as a source for $ONOO^-$ formation, but that the latter is definitely the most-important effector molecule in tissue damage. $ONOO^-$ activity, as reflected by the presence of NT, is colocalized in microglia/macrophages (which confirms the important role of these cells) and correlates with the onset of progressive clinical symptoms [47]. Upregulation of iNOS mRNA has been demonstrated in CNS of mice with EAE [48].

The first reported attempt to reduce the ROS toxicity in EAE used an iron-chelating agent, desferoxamine B mesylate (Desferal). Administration via an osmotic pump implanted subcutaneously prevented actively but not passively induced EAE in rats, and suppressed both the severity and duration of disease when administered after onset of clinical signs [49]. This protective effect may result from the removal of loosely bound iron supposed to play a role in lymphocyte recirculation and homing. A more-likely mechanism would be the chelation of free iron catalyzing the production of OH• from H_2O_2 and O_2 in activated macrophages. Administration of EUK-8, a synthetic compound displaying both SOD and catalase activities, resulted in marked amelioration of EAE disease [50].

Prevention of EAE by targeting RNS was first reported using aminoguanidine as a selective but weak inhibitor of iNOS, and was found effective to delay EAE onset and to lower the mean clinical score [51]. Pathological studies revealed a marked reduction in demyelination and axonal destruction with high doses. These beneficial effects were confirmed using the same experimental protocol [52]. In contrast, another study testing four L-arginine analogue iNOS inhibitors did not show any beneficial effect. Methodological differences may explain this disparity [53].

To interfere with nitrogen products involved at different steps in the RNS pathway, three compounds were tested in acute EAE [54]: tricyclodecan-9-yl-xanthogenate was used as an inhibitor of iNOS induction, a carboxylated derivative of 2-phenyl-tetramethylimidazoline oxyl-oxide as a NO• scavenger, and trihydroxypurine (uric acid) as a scavenger of $ONOO^-$. All tested molecules proved to be effective, but a complete protection was obtained with uric acid only.

A further study [55] focused on uric acid efficacy administered after onset of symptoms and in chronic EAE. Uric acid treatment initiated 12 days after immunization provides a dramatic improvement in animals already deteriorating. Discontinuation of the treatment leads to a reactivation of the disease after 4 days. Given the rapid metabolism of uric acid, the best clinical outcomes were obtained with four daily doses. In IFN-γ R KO mice with a severe progressive disease, four daily doses beginning 19 days after immunization delayed the onset and reduced the severity of clinical signs.

Prevention of Oxidative Stress in MS

The first clinical trial to reverse oxidative mechanisms in MS patients used antioxidant supplementation (selenium). The biochemical abnormalities reflecting an increased oxidative metabolism were reversed, but clinical effects were not reported [19]. In 1989, a trial with an iron chelating agent (Desferal) in 12 secondary progressive MS patients with a severe disability found that it was well tolerated, but no long-term clinical benefit was reported [56].

Given the significant therapeutic value of uric acid in EAE, it was suggested that this molecule might play a role in MS [55]. Significantly lower serum levels of uric acid were found in MS patients and it was hypothesized that they reflected an inadequate protection against $ONOO^-$ damage associated with MS acute progression. Interestingly, an epidemiological study revealed that the prevalence of MS is markedly lower than expected in patients with gout (expected $0.03/10^5$, observed $0.002/10^5$).

Hyperuricemia was observed in MS patients after administration of isoprinosine, an immunoregulator with the potential to restore deficient immunosuppressive functions. Isoprinosine is a molecular complex of inosine and the p-acetaminobenzoic acid salt of N,N-dimethylamino-2-propanol (Pranobex) in a 1:3 molar ratio. Results from clinical studies in immunodeficient patients

[57] show that the major excretion product of isoprinosine is uric acid, which accounts for 30%-70% of the administered inosine. Administration of inoprinosine produces an elevation in serum uric acid levels that is definitely more marked in males than in females. In spite of levels that could be considered hyperuricemic, no pathological signs or symptoms were noted and the good tolerance and safety of isoprinosine was confirmed after administration for several years.

Several open clinical trials with isoprinosine were conducted in MS patients with conflicting results [58-63]. Methodological bias makes it difficult to evaluate a potential benefit. There were major differences between dosages, treatment regimens, patient selection and number, follow-up, etc...

More recently two placebo-controlled trials have been reported. In the study of Milligan et al. [64], 52 patients with RR and relapsing-progressing (RP) MS received isoprinosine or placebo for 2 years following a single, pulsed, intravenous administration of methylprednisolone. Due to a randomization error, more patients in the treated (17/25) than in the placebo group (9/17) had RRMS. However, both groups had a low disability level (mean EDSS RR 2.2, RP 3.6) and the relapse rate was quite similar. Comparing all patients receiving isoprinosine or placebo, no benefit was demonstrated on the relapse rate, but a definite trend in favor of isoprinosine was found concerning the percentage of patients with progression, as reflected by EDSS and ambulation index increase (isoprinosine 21%, placebo 48%). This trend was even more pronounced in RP patients (isoprinosine 14%, placebo 61%).

The Isoprinosine European Study, presented at the 9th ECTRIMS Congress [65], was a randomized, double-blind, placebo-controlled trial including 97 patients with RRMS (mean annual relapse rate, treated 1.70 ± 0.4, placebo 1.65 ± 0.4; mean EDSS, treated 3.14 ± 1.56, placebo 2.91 ± 1.50). After 2 years, no significant benefit on the relapse rate or on the mean EDSS was observed, but the treatment failure (TF) (EDSS ≥ 1 confirmed at 3 months) revealed a significant benefit in the isoprinosine group: TF isoprinosine 17.65% versus TF placebo 39.16% (log rank test $p=0.04$). This difference between the two groups is mainly due to a better response in female patients [TF isoprinosine 15.15% versus TF placebo 37.98% ($p=0.07$)] compared with male patients: TF isoprinosine 22.22% versus placebo 41.48% ($p=0.33$)]. However, given the small number of patients in both subgroups, this benefit is not statistically significant.

This disparity between therapeutic responses correlated with sex differences in mean serum uric acid levels not only at baseline (males 4.35 ± 1.07 mg/dl, females 3.48 ± 0.99 mg/dl) but also after administration of isoprinosine (males 6.18 ± 1.58 mg/dl, females 4.00 ± 1.14 mg/dl).

Differences in the metabolism of uric acid between male and female populations have been reported. In healthy people, the mean serum uric acid level is lower in females than in males [66], and after administration of inosine, serum uric acid is significantly lower in females, suggesting a different metabolism of uric acid in women [57, 67].

Attention has recently focused on the potential role of uric acid in MS. Lower serum uric acid levels were found in relapsing versus stable patients, and a decrease in these levels during relapses was demonstrated with serial analyses [68]. Lower serum uric acid levels have been reported in type 1 diabetic patients, another autoimmune disease [69]. A significant increase in serum uric acid levels was observed after administration of glatiramer acetate in MS patients, but not after IFNβ-1a treatment, suggesting that uric acid production might be one of the mechanisms of action of glatiramer acetate [70].

Oxidative Mechanisms as a Therapeutic Target in MS

Oxidative mechanisms certainly play a role in MS and experimental as well as pathological observations of MS plaques demonstrate that oxidative toxicity is definitely more involved in active than in chronic MS lesions. Consequently, patients with a RRMS would likely benefit the most from antioxidant therapy.

ROS, and particularly OH•, do not seem to play a major role in MS pathophysiology, but RNS are definitely of major concern. The basic reaction occurs between NO• and O_2^-, forming $ONOO^-$ that decomposes into nitrate (an inert product) and into reactive intermediates mediating oxidative (proteins, lipids, and nucleic acid) as well as nitration and nitrosation reactions.

A first therapeutic approach would be the control of $ONOO^-$ formation with NO•, O_2^-, or iNOS-specific scavengers or inhibitors. Most results in EAE are conflicting and demonstrate a moderate efficacy only. Interestingly, in recent experiments, neither NO• nor O_2^- alone induced lipid peroxidation, which was actually inhibited by NO•. $ONOO^-$ formation seems thus required for myelin-lipid peroxidation [71].

A second approach is a direct reaction with $ONOO^-$, blocking its further degradation or leading to non-toxic products. In recent years, numerous scavengers have been found effective to protect in a catalytic fashion against $ONOO^-$ toxicity in vitro: uric acid [72], tirilazad mesylate [73], several antibiotics [74], ergothioneine [75], 21-aminosteroids [76], L-ascorbic acid [77], melatonin [78], selenoproteins (Ebselen) [79-81], tellurides [82], natural sulfur compound (AECK) [83], mercaptoethylguanidine [84, 85], metalloporphyrins [86, 87], hydroxycinnamate [88], glutathione peroxidase [89], and N-acetylcysteine [90].

$ONOO^-$ can also elicit both apoptosis and necrosi in cell culture. Prevention has been demonstrated with an inhibitor (INH2BP) of a nuclear enzyme (poly-ADP-ribose) [91, 92], with a new derivative of vitamin C and E (EPC-K1) [93], with nerve growth factor [94], with cycloheximide (Deprenyl) [95], and by blocking exocytosis with tetanus toxin or botulism neurotoxin C [96].

A third avenue would be the use of scavengers of secondary oxidants formed by $ONOO^-$. So far only bilirubin [97] and aminoguanidine [98] have been reported to be effective, apparently by this mechanism. It is noteworthy that several recent publications demonstrate the inhibitory effects of IFN-β on two oxidative mechanisms: iNOS [99, 100] and ROS production [101].

Uric Acid: a Potential Antioxidant to Delay Progression in RRMS?

Among several molecules tested in EAE, uric acid seems the most efficient [55]. Uric acid is a well-known natural antioxidant operating by different mechanisms: suppression of accumulation of H_2O_2 and $ONOO^-$, stabilization of intracellular calcium homeostasis, and preservation of mitochondrial function [102]. Its efficacy is clearly dose dependent [103, 104].

Oral administration of uric acid to MS patients does not raise serum levels, probably due to its destruction by gut microbial flora [105]. Inosine, a naturally occurring substance found in the metabolic pathway of purines, is rapidly catabolyzed and its major excretion product is uric acid. Inosine has been used pre heavy training by athletes. Its daily administration (5-6 g) did not improve aerobic performances, but was well tolerated despite a significant hyperuricemia [106]. Interestingly, inosine has been found to be effective recently to prevent astroglial injuries in vitro during combined O_2^- glucose deprivation [107], to protect against neuronal necrosis observed under experimental hypoxic conditions [108], to promote axon outgrowth in vitro and in vivo after corticospinal tract transection [109, 110], and to inhibit inflammatory cytokine production [111].

It has been shown recently [105] that daily oral administration of inosine to MS patients leads to elevated serum uric acid levels (approximately 7-8 g/dl). This hyperuricemia was maintained for 1 year without any adverse reaction. In the European Isoprinosine Study, the mean serum uric acid level was increased from 3.70 ± 1.17 g/dl to 5.11 ± 1.59 g/dl ($p = 0.005$).

Since demyelination and axonal loss involve the cooperation of both immune-mediated inflammatory mechanisms and oxidative mechanisms, new therapeutic efforts associating an anti-inflammatory drug (IFN-β) and an antioxidative molecule (inosine, an inexpensive and non-toxic natural metabolite) appear warranted. This combined therapy might delay the transition from the RR to the progressive phase more efficiently than with IFNs alone.

Treatment of Early Disability Due to Frequent and Disabling Relapses

During the RR phase, some patients experience severe and frequent relapses, accumulating neurological sequelae and leading to an early development of disability. Mitoxantrone (MX) is a broad immunosuppressor with an impact not only on the cellular components but mainly on the humoral components of the immune system. It inhibits antibody production by B cells and blocks demyelinating activity of macrophages [112]. Given the crucial role of macrophages in MS pathogenesis, as well as their close interaction with oxidative mechanisms, it was likely that a drug specifically inhibiting their activity would have a beneficial effect on disease progression [113]. It was soon observed that MX also had a potent anti-inflammatory activity demonstrated by the rapid abrogation of gadolinium (Gd)-enhancing lesions in treated patients [114, 115]. The study of Edan et al. [116] demonstrated that intensive immunotherapy with MX is able to block the dramatic evolution in most patients. The clinical characteristics of those patients are a young age (30 ± 10 years), a short duration of disease (6 ± 4 years), and a low EDSS (4 ± 1). They experience at least two relapses per year without complete recovery, leading to a rapid progression of the disease, as reflected by an increase of ≥ 2 points on the EDSS scale over 1 year. Magnetic resonance imaging (MRI) demonstrates numerous Gd-enhancing lesions, indicating major focal inflammatory reactions.

Several arguments suggest that to obtain an early and durable benefit a treatment combining an induction phase followed by a maintenance phase would be the most-appropriate regimen. The rationale for an induction phase relies on the presence of very active inflammatory reactions in those patients and the need to rapidly control the disease progression. A recent study with cyclophosphamide [117] demonstrates that the best benefit is obtained after a short-term intensive induction phase followed by 2-monthly administration, compared with boosters given straight-away every 2 months. In addition, the rationale for a preliminary induction phase is supported by MRI demonstrating that eradication of Gd-enhancing lesions with monthly administration occurs after 2 months [116], and after 6 months only with quarterly administration [115].

The most-effective dose for MX administration seems to be 12 mg/m². Given the frequent dosage adjustments, the cumulative dose over 2 years treatment would be about 100 mg/m², definitely within the safety limits for cardiotoxicity (recommended maximum cumulative dose 120 mg/m²).

Conclusions

Current data concerning the role of oxidative mechanisms during the RR phase, animal experiments, and preliminary clinical trials suggest that a combined therapy with anti-inflammatory drugs (IFN-β) and antioxidants (uric acid) might delay the transition to the progressive phase more efficiently than anti-inflammatory drugs alone.

The protocol of a clinical trial (Association of Inosine and Interferon-β in Relapsing-Remitting Multiple Sclerosis, ASIIMS study) is underway. In patients with RRMS with an acute progression leading to the development of an early disability, a proper administration of MX has proven able to abrogate associated acute inflammatory processes and stabilize most patients. A treatment period of 2 years combining an induction and a maintenance phase seems the most-appropriate regimen.

References

1. Raine CS (1994) The Dale E. McFarlin memorial lecture: the immunology of the multiple sclerosis lesion. Ann Neurol 36:S61-S72
2. Trapp BD, Ransohoff RM, Fisher E, Rudick RA (1999) Neurodegeneration in multiple sclerosis: relationship to neurological disability. Neuroscientist 5:48-57

3. Smith KJ, Kapoor R, Felts PA (1999) Demyelination: the role of reactive oxygen and nitrogen species. Brain Pathol 9:69-92
4. Redford EJ, Kapoor R, Smith KJ (1997) Nitric oxide donors reversibly block axonal conduction: demyelinated axons are especially susceptible. Brain 120:2149-2157
5. Kapoor R, Davies M, Smith KJ (1999) Temporary axonal conduction block and axonal loss in inflammatory neurological disease. A potential role for nitric oxide? Ann NY Acad Sci 893:304-308
6. Kim YS, Kim SU (1991) Oligodendroglial cell death induced by oxygen radicals and its protection by catalase. J Neurosci Res 29:100-106
7. Merrill JE et al (1993) Microglial cell cytotoxicity of oligodendrocytes is mediated through nitric oxide. J Immunol 151:2132-2141
8. Mitrovic B et al (1995) Nitric oxide induces necrotic but not apoptotic cell death in oligodendrocytes. Neuroscience 65:531-539
9. Mickel HS (1975) Multiple sclerosis: a new hypothesis. Perspect Biol Med 18:363-374
10. Reif DW, Simmons RD (1990) Nitric oxide mediates iron release from ferritin. Arch Biochem Biophys 283:537-541
11. Beckman JS (1994) Peroxynitrite versus hydroxyl radical: the role of nitric oxide in superoxide-dependent cerebral injury. Ann NY Acad Sci 738:69-75
12. Le Vine SM (1992) The role of reactive oxygen species in the pathogenesis of multiple sclerosis. Med Hypotheses 39:271-274
13. Kolb H, Kolb-Bachofen V (1992) Nitric oxide: a pathogenetic factor in autoimmunity. Immunol Today 13:157-159
14. Brosnan CF et al (1994) Reactive nitrogen intermediates in human neuropathology: an overview. Dev Neurosci 16:152-161
15. Molina JA, Jimenez-Jimenez FJ, Orti-Pareja M, Navarro JA (1998) The role of nitric oxide in neurodegeneration. Potential for pharmacological intervention. Drugs Aging 12:251-259
16. Beckman JS, Koppenol WH (1996) Nitric oxide, superoxide, and peroxynitrite: the good, the bad, and the ugly. Am J Physiol 271:C1424-C1437
17. Lorsbach RB et al (1993) Expression of the nitric oxide synthase gene in mouse macrophages activated for tumor cell killing. J Biol Chem 268:1908-1913
18. Mazella GL et al (1983) Blood cells glutathione peroxidase activity and selenium in multiple sclerosis. Eur Neurol 22:442-446
19. Jensen GE, Clausen J (1986) Glutathione peroxidase activity, associated enzymes and substrates in blood cells from patients with multiple sclerosis – effects of antioxidant supplementation. Acta Pharmacol Toxicol 59 [Suppl 7]:450-453
20. Hammann KP, Hopf HC (1986) Monocytes constitute the only peripheral blood cell population showing an increased burst activity in multiple sclerosis patients. Int Arch Allergy Appl Immun 81:230-234
21. Fisher M et al (1988) Monocyte and polymorphonuclear leukocyte toxic oxygen metabolite production in multiple sclerosis. Inflammation 12:123-131
22. Korpela H et al (1989) Serum selenium concentration, glutathione peroxidase activity and lipid peroxides in a co-twin control study on multiple sclerosis. J Neurol Sci 91:79-84
23. Glabinski A, Tawsek NS, Bartosz G (1993) Increased generation of superoxide radicals in the blood of MS patients. Acta Neurol Scand 88:174-177
24. Zabaleta ME, Bianco NE, De Sanctis JB (1998) Serum nitric oxide products in patients with multiple sclerosis: relationship with clinical activity. Med Sci Res 26:373-374
25. Giovannoni G et al (1997) Raised serum nitrate and nitrite levels in patients with multiple sclerosis. J Neurol Sci 145:77-81
26. Giovannoni G (1998) Cerebrospinal fluid and serum nitric oxide metabolites in patients with multiple sclerosis. Mult Scler 4:27-30

27. Brundin L et al (1998) Nitric oxide production in multiple sclerosis – an indicator of active disease. Mult Scler 4:327
28. Zabaleta ME, Bianco NE, De Sanctis JB (1998) Serum nitrotyrosine levels in patients with multiple sclerosis: relationship with clinical activity. Med Sci Res 26:407-408
29. Boullerne AI, Petry KG, Meynard M, Geffard M (1995) Indirect evidence for nitric oxide involvement in multiple sclerosis by characterization of circulating antibodies directed against conjugated S-nitrosocysteine. J Neuroimmunol 60:117-124
30. Karg E et al (1999) Nonenzymatic antioxidants of blood in multiple sclerosis. J Neurol 246:533-539
31. Lucas M et al (1999) The oxidation-reduction state of serum proteins in multiple sclerosis patients: effect of interferon beta-1b. Neurochem Int 34:287-289
32. Hunter MIS, Nlemadim BC, Davidson DLW (1985) Lipid peroxidation products and antioxidant proteins in plasma and cerebrospinal fluid from multiple sclerosis patients. Neurochem Res 10:1645-1652
33. Johnson AW et al (1995) Evidence for increased nitric oxide production in multiple sclerosis. J Neurol Neurosurg Psychiatry 58:107
34. Yamashita T et al (1997) Changes in nitrite and nitrate (NO2-/NO3-) levels in cerebrospinal fluid of patients with multiple sclerosis. J Neurol Sci 153:32-34
35. Svenningsson A, Petersson AS, Andersen O, Hansson GK (1999) Nitric oxide metabolites in CSF of patients with MS are related to clinical disease course. Neurology 53:1880-1882
36. De Bustos F et al (1999) Cerebrospinal fluid nitrate levels in patients with multiple sclerosis. Eur Neurol 41:44-47
37. Drulovic J et al (2001) Raised cerebrospinal fluid nitrite and nitrate levels in patients with multiple sclerosis: no correlation with disease activity. Mult Scler 7:19-22
38. Greco A et al (1999) Cerebrospinal fluid isoprostane shows oxidative stress in patients with multiple sclerosis. Neurology 53:1876-1879
39. Langemann H, Kabiersch A, Newcombe J (1992) Measurement of low-molecular-weight antioxidants, uric acid, tyrosine and tryptophan in plaques and white matter from patients with multiple sclerosis. Eur Neurol 32:248-252
40. Bö L et al (1994) Induction of nitric oxide synthase in demyelinating regions of multiple sclerosis brains. Ann Neurol 36:778-786
41. De Groot CJA et al (1997) Immunocytochemical characterization of the expression of inducible and constitutive isoforms of nitric oxide synthase in demyelinating multiple sclerosis lesions. J Neuropathol Exp Neurol 56:10-20
42. Oleszak EL et al (1998) Inducible nitric oxide synthase and nitrotyrosine are found in monocytes/macrophages and/or astrocytes in acute, but not in chronic, multiple sclerosis. Clin Diagn Lab Immunol 5:438-445
43. Cross AH et al (1998) Peroxynitrite formation within the central nervous system in active multiple sclerosis. J Neuroimmunol 88:45-56
44. Vladimirova O et al (1998) Oxidative damage to DNA in plaques of MS brains. Mult Scler 4:413-418
45. Le Vine SM, Wetzel DL (1998) Chemical analysis of multiple sclerosis lesions by FT-IR microspectroscopy. Free Radic Biol Med 25:33-41
46. Bagasra O et al (1995) Activation of the inducible form of nitric oxide synthase in the brains of patients with multiple sclerosis. Proc Natl Acad Sci U S A 92:12041-12045
47. Van der Veen RC, Hinton DC, Incardonna F, Hofman FM (1997) Extensive peroxynitrite activity during progressive stages of central nervous system inflammation. J Neuroimmunol 77:1-7
48. Tran EH, Hardin-Pouzet H, Verge G, Owens T (1997) Astrocytes and microglia express inducible nitric oxide synthase in mice with experimental allergic encephalomyelitis. J Neuroimmunol 74:121-129

49. Bowern N, Ramshaw IA, Clark IA, Doherty PC (1984) Inhibition of autoimmune neuropathological process by treatment with an iron-chelating agent. J Exp Med 160:1532-1543

50. Malfroy B et al (1997) Prevention and suppression of autoimmune encephalomyelitis by EUK-8, a synthetic catalytic scavenger of oxygen-reactive metabolites. Cell Immunol 177:62-68

51. Cross AH et al (1994) Aminoguanidine, an inhibitor of inducible nitric oxide synthase, ameliorates experimental autoimmune encephalomyelitis in SJL mice. J Clin Invest 93:2684-2690

52. Brenner T et al (1997) Inhibition of nitric oxide synthase for treatment of experimental autoimmune encephalomyelitis. J Immunol 158:2940-2946

53. Zielasek J et al (1995) Administration of nitric oxide synthase inhibitors in experimental autoimmune neuritis and experimental autoimmune encephalomyelitis. J Neuroimmunol 58:81-88

54. Hooper DC et al (1997) Prevention of experimental allergic encephalomyelitis by targeting nitric oxide and peroxynitrite: implications for the treatment of multiple sclerosis. Proc Natl Acad Sci U S A 94:2528-2533

55. Hooper DC et al (1998) Uric acid, a natural scavenger of peroxynitrite, in experimental allergic encephalomyelitis and multiple sclerosis. Proc Natl Acad Sci U S A 95:675-680

56. Norstrand IF, Craellus W (1989) A trial of deferoxamine (Desferal) in the treatment of multiple sclerosis. A pilot study. Clin Trials J 26:365-369

57. Gordon J, Ginsberg T (1988) Isoprinosine and NPT 15392: hypoxanthine-containing immunomodulators. In: Bray MA (ed) Handbook of experimental pharmacology, vol 85. Springer, Berlin Heidelberg New York, pp 535-553

58. Mazzarello P et al (1982) Isoprinosine in multiple sclerosis treatment: a preliminary study. Arch Suisses Neurol Neurochir Psychiatry 131:175-179

59. Caltagirone C, Carlesimo A (1986) Methisoprinol in the treatment of multiple sclerosis. A pilot study. Acta Neurol Scand 74:293-296

60. Pompidou A et al (1986) Clinical and immunological improvement of remittent multiple sclerosis after treatment with isoprinosine. A randomized pilot study. Presse Med 15:930-931

61. Pompidou A et al (1987) Immunosuppressive effects of isoprinosine in man: a comparison to chlorambucil effects in multiple sclerosis. Cancer Detect Prev [Suppl] 1:377-383

62. Confavreux C et al (1986) Treatment of multiple sclerosis with isoprinosine. 52 observations. Presse Med 15:2256-2257

63. Maciejek Z (1989) Changes in visual evoked potentials in patients with multiple sclerosis treated with isoprinosine and amantadine. Arch Immunol Ther Exp 37:621-628

64. Milligan NM, Miller DH, Compston DAS (1994) A placebo-controlled trial of isoprinosine in patients with multiple sclerosis. J Neurol Neurosurg Psychiatry 57:164-168

65. Gonsette RE et al (1993) The European Isoprinosine Study in Multiple Sclerosis (abstract). ECTRIMS AISM Congress Florence, 31 October to 2 November, p 50

66. Alderman MH, Cohen H, Madhavan S, Kivlighn S (1999) Serum uric acid and cardiovascular events in successfully treated hypertensive patients. Hypertension 34:144-150

67. Wicket WH et al (1984) A double-blinded study of medium to long-term safety of inosiplex in the treatment of recurrent genital herpes virus disease. Curr Ther Res 35:177-183

68. Drulovic J et al (2001) Uric acid levels in sera from patients with multiple sclerosis. J Neurol 248:121-126

69. Zazgornik J et al (1996) Serum uric acid level in type 1 and type 2 diabetic patients. Wien Med Wochenschr 146:102-104

70. Constantinescu CS, Freitag P, Kappos L (2000) Increase of serum levels of uric acid, an endogenous antioxidant, under treatment with glatiramer acetate for multiple sclerosis. Mult Scler 6:378-381

71. Van der Veen RC, Roberts LJ (1999) Contrasting roles for nitric oxide and peroxynitrite in the peroxidation of myelin lipids. J Neuroimmunol 95:1-7

72. Whiteman M, Halliwell B (1996) Protection against peroxynitrite-dependent tyrosine nitration and alpha 1-antiproteinase inactivation by ascorbic acid. A comparison with other biological antioxidants. Free Radic Res 25:275-283

73. Fici GJ, Althaus JS, Hall ED, Von Voigtlander PF (1996) Protective effects of tirilazad mesylate in a cellular model of peroxynitrite toxicity. Res Commun Mol Pathol Pharmacol 91:357-371

74. Whiteman M, Halliwell B (1997) Prevention of peroxynitrite-dependent tyrosine nitration and inactivation of alpha1-antiproteinase by antibiotics. Free Radic Res 26:49-56

75. Aruoma OI, Whiteman M, England TG, Halliwell B (1997) Antioxidant action of ergothioneine: assessment of its ability to scavenge peroxynitrite. Biochem Biophys Res Commun 231:389-391

76. Fici GJ, Althaus JS, Von Voigtlander PF (1997) Effects of lazaroids and a peroxynitrite scavenger in a cell model of peroxynitrite toxicity. Free Radic Biol Med 22:223-228

77. Sandoval M et al (1997) Peroxynitrite-induced apoptosis in T84 and RAW 264.7 cells: attenuation by L-ascorbic acid. Free Radic Biol Med 22:489-495

78. Gilad E et al (1997) Melatonin is a scavenger of peroxynitrite. Life Sci 60:169-174

79. Sies H et al (1998) Protection against peroxynitrite by selenoproteins. Z Naturforsch [C]53:228-232

80. Masumoto H, Kissner R, Koppenol WH, Sies H (1996) Kinetic study of the reaction of ebselen with peroxynitrite. FEBS Lett 398:179-182

81. Ducrocq C, Blanchard B, Pignatelli B, Ohshima H (1998) Oxidative chemistry of nitric oxide: the roles of superoxide, peroxynitrite, and carbon dioxide. Free Radic Biol Med 55:392-403

82. Briviba K et al (1998) Protection by organotellurium compounds against peroxynitrite-mediated oxidation and nitration reactions. Biochem Pharmacol 55:817-823

83. Fontana M, Pecci L, Macone A, Cavallini D (1998) Antioxidant properties of the decarboxylated dimer of aminoethylcysteine ketimine: assessment of its ability to scavenge peroxynitrite. Free Radic Res 29:435-440

84. Cuzzocrea S et al (1998) Antiinflammatory effects of mercaptoethylguanidine, a combined inhibitor of nitric oxide synthase and peroxynitrite scavenger, in carrageenan-induced models of inflammation. Free Radic Biol Med 24:450-459

85. Zingarelli B, Cuzzocrea S, Szab'o C, Salzman AL (1998) Mercaptoethylguanidine, a combined inhibitor of nitric oxide synthase and peroxynitrite scavenger, reduces trinitrobenzene sulfonic acid-induced colonic damage in rats. J Pharmacol Exp Ther 287:1048-1055

86. Crow JP (1999) Manganese and iron porphyrins catalyze peroxynitrite decomposition and simultaneously increase nitration and oxidant yield: implications for their use as peroxynitrite scavengers in vivo. Arch Biochem Biophys 371:41-52

87. Misko TP et al (1998) Characterization of the cytoprotective action of peroxynitrite decomposition catalysts. J Biol Chem 273:15646-15653

88. Pannala AS et al (1998) Inhibition of peroxynitrite dependent tyrosine nitration by hydroxycinnamates: nitration of electron donation? Free Radic Biol Med 24:594-606

89. Arteel GE, Briviba K, Sies H (1999) Protection against peroxynitrite. FEBS Lett 445:226-230

90. Cuzzocrea S, Costantino G, Caputi AP (1999) Protective effect of N-acetylcysteine on cellular energy depletion in non-septic shock model induced by zymosan in the rat. Shock 11:143-148

91. Szab'o C et al (1998) Protection against peroxynitrite-induced fibroblast injury and arthritis development by inhibition of poly(ADP-ribose) synthase. Proc Natl Acad Sci U S A 95:3867-3872

92. Endres M et al (1998) Protective effects of 5-iodo-6-amino-1,2-benzopyrone, an inhibitor of poly(ADP-ribose) synthetase against peroxynitrite-induced glial damage and stroke development. Eur J Pharmacol 351:377-382

93. Wei T et al (1998) EPC-K1 attenuates peroxynitrite-induced apoptosis in cerebellar granule cells. Biochem Mol Biol Int 46:89-97

94. Spear N et al (1997) Nerve growth factor protects PC12 cells against peroxynitrite-induced apoptosis via a mechanism dependent on phosphatidylinositol 3-kinase. J Neurochem 69:53-59

95. Maruyama W, Takahashi T, Naoi M (1998) (-)-Deprenyl protects human dopaminergic neuroblastoma SH-SY5Y cells from apoptosis induced by peroxynitrite and nitric oxide. J Neurochem 70:2510-2515

96. Leist M, Fava E, Montecucco C, Nicotera P (1997) Peroxynitrite and nitric oxide donors induce neuronal apoptosis by eliciting autocrine excitotoxicity. Eur J Neurosci 9:1488-1498

97. Minetti M, Mallozzi C, Di Stasi AM, Pietraforte D (1998) Bilirubin is an effective antioxidant of peroxynitrite-mediated protein oxidation in human blood plasma. Arch Biochem Biophys 352:165-174

98. Szab'o C et al (1997) Mercaptoethylguanidine and guanidine inhibitors of nitric-oxide synthase react with peroxynitrite and protect against peroxynitrite-induced oxidative damage. J Biol Chem 272:9030-9036

99. Hua LL, Liu JSH, Brosnan CF, Lee SC (1998) Selective inhibition of human glial inducible nitric oxide synthase by interferon-b: Implications for multiple sclerosis. Ann Neurol 48:384-387

100. Guthikonda P, Baker J, Mattson DH (1998) Interferon-beta-1-b (IFN-B) decreases induced nitric oxide (NO) production by a human astrocytoma cell line. J Neuroimmunol 82:133-139

101. Lucas M, Sanchez-Solino O, Solano F, Izquierdo G (1998) Interferon beta-1b inhibits reactive oxygen species production in peripheral blood monocytes of patients with relapsing-remitting multiple sclerosis. Neurochem Int 33:101-102

102. Yu ZF, Bruce-Keller AJ, Goodman Y, Mattson MP (1998) Uric acid protects neurons against excitotoxic and metabolic insults in cell culture, and against focal ischemic brain injury in vivo. J Neurosci Res 53:613-625

103. Schlotte V, Sevanian A, Hochstein P, Weithmann KU (1998) Effect of uric acid and chemical analogues on oxidation of human low density lipoprotein in vitro. Free Radic Biol Med 25:839-847

104. Halcak L, Rendekova V, Pechan I, Kubaska M (1998) The effect of uric acid, creatine phosphate and carnitine on lipid peroxidation in cerebral cortex and myocardium homogenates. Bratisl Lek Listy 99:343-346

105. Koprowski H, Spitsin SV, Hooper DC (2001) Prospects for the treatment of multiple sclerosis by raising serum levels of uric acid, a scavenger of peroxynitrite. Ann Neurol 49:139

106. Starling RD et al (1996) Effect of inosine supplementation on aerobic and anaerobic cycling performance. Med Sci Sports Exerc 28:1193-1198

107. Haun SE et al (1996) Inosine mediates the protective effect of adenosine in rat astrocyte cultures subjected to combined glucose-oxygen deprivation. J Neurochem 67:2051-2059

108. Litsky ML, Hohl CM, Lucas JH, Jurkowitz MS (1999) Inosine and guanosine preserve neuronal and glial cell viability in mouse spinal cord cultures during chemical hypoxia. Brain Res 821:426-432

109. Benowitz LI et al (1999) Inosine stimulates extensive axon collateral growth in the rat corticospinal tract after injury. Proc Natl Acad Sci U S A 96:13486-13490

110. Hadlock T et al (1999) A novel, biodegradable polymer conduit delivers neurotrophins and promotes nerve regeneration. Laryngoscope 109:1412-1416
111. Hasko G et al (2000) Inosine inhibits inflammatory cytokine production by a post-transcriptional mechanism and protects against endotoxin-induced shock. J Immunol 164:1013-1019
112. Watson CM et al (1991) Suppression of demyelination by mitoxantrone. Int J Immunopharmacal 13:923-930
113. Gonsette RE, Demonty L (1989) Mitoxantrone: a new immunosuppressive agent in multiple sclerosis. In: Gonsette RE, Delmotte P (eds) Recent advances in multiple sclerosis therapy. Elsevier Science, Amsterdam, pp 161-164
114. Kappos L et al (1990) Mitoxantrone (Mx) in the treatment of rapidly progressive MS: A pilot study with serial gadolinium (Gd)-enhanced MRI. Neurology 40 [Suppl] 1:261
115. Krapf H et al (1995) Serial gadolinium-enhanced magnetic resonance imaging in patients with multiple sclerosis treated with mitoxantrone. Neuroradiology 37:113-119
116. Edan G et al (1997) Therapeutic effect of mitoxantrone combined with methylprednisolone in multiple sclerosis: a randomised multicentre study of active disease using MRI and clinical criteria. J Neurol Neurosurg Psychiatry 62:112-118
117. La Mantia L et al (1998) Cyclophosphamide in chronic progressive multiple sclerosis: a comparative study. Ital J Neurol Sci 19:32-36

Imaging for Tissue Characterization in Multiple Sclerosis and Other White Matter Diseases

M. Filippi, N. De Stefano

Introduction

In white matter diseases (WMD), conventional magnetic resonance imaging (MRI) has proved to be sensitive for detecting lesions and their changes over time. However, conventional MRI is not able to characterize and quantify the tissue damage within and outside these lesions. Other quantitative MR techniques have the potential to overcome such limitation. Among these techniques, MR spectroscopy (MRS), magnetization transfer imaging (MTI), and diffusion-weighted imaging (DWI) have been most extensively applied to the assessment of WMD. The present review will summarize the major contributions of these three MR techniques to the understanding of the evolution of WMD, with a special focus on multiple sclerosis (MS). The application of MR techniques to the study of MS has indeed dramatically changed our understanding of how MS causes irreversible deficits and can serve as a useful model to be applied to other WMD.

Magnetic Resonance Spectroscopy

MRS techniques can complement conventional MRI in the assessment of patients with WMD by defining simultaneously several chemical correlates of the pathological changes occurring within and outside T2-visible lesions. Water-suppressed, proton MR spectra of normal human brain at long echo times reveal four major resonances: one at 3.2 ppm from tetramethylamines [mainly from choline-containing phospholipids (Cho)], one at 3.0 ppm from creatine and phosphocreatine (Cr), one at 2.0 ppm from *N*-acetyl groups [mainly *N*-acetyl aspartate (NAA)], and one at 1.3 ppm from the methyl resonance of lactate (Lac). Although more technically demanding, additional metabolites [including lipids and *myo*-inositol (mI)] can be detected in WMD using short echo time measurements.

Proton MRS of acute MS lesions at both short and long echo times reveals increases in Cho and Lac resonance intensities from the early phases of the pathological process [1, 2]. Changes in the resonance intensity of Cho result mainly from increases in the steady-state levels of phosphocholine and glycerol phosphocholine, both membrane phospholipids that are released during active myelin breakdown. Increases in Lac are likely to reflect the metabolism of inflammatory cells. In large, acute demyelinating lesions, decreases of Cr can also be seen [2]. Short echo time spectra give evidence for transient increases in visible lipids, released during myelin breakdown, and mI [1, 3]. All these changes are usually followed by a decrease in NAA. Since NAA is a metabolite detected only in neurons and their processes in normal mature brains, the decrease in NAA is presumably secondary to axonal dysfunction. After the acute phase and over a period of days to weeks, there is a progressive reduction of raised Lac resonance intensities to normal levels. Resonance intensities of Cr also return to normal within a few days. Cho, lipid, and mI resonance intensities return to normal over months. The signal intensity of NAA may remain decreased or show partial recovery, starting soon after the acute phase and lasting for several months [1, 4, 5]. Recovery of NAA may be related to resolution of edema, increases in the diameter of previously shrunk axons secondary to remyelination, and clearance of inflammatory factors and reversible metabolic changes in neurons. Although similar decreases in NAA are found in acute enhancing lesions of patients with benign and secondary progressive MS (SPMS), chronic lesions from patients with benign MS have much higher NAA levels than the chronic lesions from SPMS patients, suggesting a greater recovery of NAA in acute lesions from less-disabled MS patients [6]. Since in acute MS lesions gadolinium enhancement usually ceases by 2 months, the metabolic changes shown by MRS techniques can reveal on-going pathology relevant for determining the clinical manifestations of the disease, but which would otherwise go undetected. Interestingly, a recent study detected elevated lipid peaks also in regions of normal-appearing white matter (NAWM). In some of these regions, this MRS abnormality preceded new MS lesion formation [3].

Since changes in axonal viability may be important determinants of functional impairment in MS, one of the major contributions of MRS to the understanding of MS is likely to be the quantification of axonal pathology, by measuring NAA levels in lesions and NAWM. The importance of axonal damage in determining clinical deficits in MS has been shown by several authors [4, 5-7]. The most-elegant study is by Davie et al. [8], who found reduced cerebellar NAA levels in patients with MS and cerebellar ataxia, similar to that present in those with autosomal dominant spinocerebellar degeneration. The levels of cerebellar NAA were normal in non-ataxic MS patients. The magnitude of the generalized decrease in brain NAA can be estimated using a single large voxel centered on the corpus callosum. Decreased NAA levels are found in patients with established MS from the early phases of the disease [4, 5]. Although the extent of the decrease in NAA per unit lesion volume is greater in SPMS than in relapsing-remitting MS (RRMS), the rate of NAA change with time is faster in RRMS than in SPMS [9]. Strong inverse correlations between NAA and disability levels have been found in patients with isolated acute demyelinating lesions [2] and in patients with RRMS [10]. A weaker, but significant correlation has also been found in patients with SPMS [10].

Decreases in NAA are not restricted to T2-visible lesions, but occur also in the NAWM adjacent to or distant from them [11]. This is consistent with post-mortem studies showing axonal loss in the NAWM of MS patients [11]. Anterograde and retrograde degeneration of axons traversing large lesions appears to be the most-likely pathological substrate, at least in patients with high lesion loads. The role of this factor in determining MRS changes in NAWM is supported by the recent finding [12] of dramatic, but reversible changes of NAA in the NAWM of the hemisphere contralateral to solitary acute MS lesions. However, small focal abnormalities independent from larger T2-visible lesions can also contribute to NAA decreases in NAWM. This seems to be the case for patients with primary progressive MS (PPMS), who have markedly reduced NAA levels in the NAWM despite the paucity of T2 abnormalities [13]. Recently, it has been shown that NAWM from SPMS patients has on average 8.2% lower NAA levels than NAWM from RRMS [14]. However, in RRMS patients a progressive reduction of NAWM NAA is detectable over time, and this decrease correlates strongly with accumulation of disability [14].

Proton MRS has also been used to assess brain pathology in patients with WMD other than MS. Brain WMD are secondary to a variety of pathological processes and are associated with many different myelin abnormalities. This heterogeneity may render the diagnostic work-up particularly challenging. Although the vast majority of the MRI and MRS changes dectected in WMD are not disease specific, the complementary information from the two techniques can significantly increase the diagnostic confidence [15]. For instance, in Canavan's disease the deficiency of the enzyme aspartoacylase results in abnormally high levels of brain NAA [16]. Leukoencephalopathy with vanishing WM can be differentiated from leukoencephalopathy with swelling by the abnormally high Lac and glucose resonance intensities found only in the former condition [17]. Brain metabolic changes seen in patients with Alzheimer disease (decreases in NAA and increases in mI and Cho) and vascular dementia (decreases in NAA) are usually not detected in mentally normal elderly subjects with leukoaraiosis [18]. MRS has also been used to increase the understanding of WMD evolution. In leukoencephalopathies, Cho, mI, and mobile lipid increases are usually seen during the early process of myelin breakdown and are interpreted as indices of active demyelination [19-21]. In slowly progressive disorders, such as many leukodystrophies, where the loss of myelin is very slow and released membrane phospholipids do not accumulate, such MRS changes are not seen [19, 20, 22, 23]. This is not the case for adrenoleukodystrophy, in which long-term increases in Cho are probably due to a high membrane turnover [22]. Decrease in Cho secondary to hypomyelination or vacuolar myelinopathy can be detected in Canavan's disease or mitochondrial disorders, respectively [15]. In patients with both hereditary and acquired leukoencephalopaties, a common MRS finding is represented by the decrease in brain NAA, which is evident both in lesions and NAWM [15, 24]. As in MS, in this heterogeneous group of disorders, NAA levels correlate well with neurological impairment, suggesting that axonal damage represents one of the substrates of functional impairment in several WMD.

Magnetization Transfer Imaging

MTI is based on the interactions between protons in a relatively free environment and those where motion is restricted. In the central nervous system (CNS), these two states correspond to the protons in tissue water, and in the macromolecules of myelin and other cell membranes. Off-resonance irradiation is applied, which saturates the magnetization of the less-mobile protons, but this is transferred to the mobile protons, thus reducing the signal intensity from the observable magnetization. The degree of signal loss depends on the density of the macromolecules in a given tissue. Thus, a low MT ratio (MTR) indicates a reduced capacity of the macromolecules in CNS tissue to exchange magnetization with the surrounding water molecules, reflecting damage to myelin or to the axonal membrane. There are several lines of evidence to suggest that a marked reduction of MTR values in MS lesions indicates severe tissue damage [25]. The most-compelling evidence comes from a recent post-mortem study showing strong correlations of MTR values from MS lesions and NAWM with the percentage of residual axons and the degree of demyelination [26].

Using MTI and variable frequencies of scanning, several authors have investigated the structural changes of new enhancing MS lesions for periods of time ranging from 3 to 36 months [25]. The results of all these studies consistently show that, on average, MTR drops dramatically when the lesions start to enhance and may show a partial or complete recovery in the subsequent one to six months. The relatively good preservation of axons that is usual in acute MS lesions, and the rapid and marked increase of the MTR, suggest demyelination and remyelination as the most-likely pathological mechanisms underlying these short-term MTR changes. Nevertheless, edema and its subsequent resolution may also give rise to the observed pattern of MTR behavior, due to the diluting effect of extra tissue water. However, it seems unlikely that edema alone is sufficient to explain these findings, since previous studies [27, 28] showed that edema in the absence of demyelination results in only modest MTR reductions. MTI studies of individual enhancing lesions also confirmed that the pathological nature of such lesions and the severity of the associated changes in the inflamed tissue may vary considerably [29-31]. These changes seem to be related to the severity [32] and duration [33] of the opening of the blood-brain barrier.

These results suggest that the balance between damaging and reparative mechanisms may be highly variable from the early phases of MS lesion formation. Different proportions of lesions with different degrees of structural changes may, therefore, contribute to the evolution of the disease. At present, however, there are few data supporting this concept. A recent 3-year follow-up study [34] showed that newly formed lesions from patients with SPMS have lower MTR and present a more-severe MTR reduction during the follow-up than those from patients with less-disabling RRMS. Consistent with MRS findings, MTR reductions can be detected in the NAWM before lesion formation [35]. Edema, marked astrocytic proliferation, perivascular inflammation, and demyelination may all account for an increased amount of unbound water in the NAWM [11] and, as a consequence, determine MTR changes.

Consistent with their pathological heterogeneity, established MS lesions have a wide range of MTR values [27, 36]. A lower MTR has been reported in hypointense lesions than in lesions that are isointense to NAWM on T1-weighted scans [30, 37], and MTR has been inversely correlated with the degree of hypointensity [30]. In a longitudinal study with monthly MTI and T1-weighted scans, van Waesberghe et al. [37] found that MS lesions that changed from hypointense to isointense when gadolinium enhancement ceased, also had a significant MTR increase, whereas a strongly decreased MTR at the time of initial enhancement was predictive of a persistent T1-weighted hypointensity and lower MTR after 6 months. Decreased MTR has also been found for NAWM from MS [38, 39], even in the absence of T2-visible lesions [40]. These changes are more pronounced in NAWM areas adjacent to focal T2-weighted MS lesions [38, 39], particularly in SPMS patients [38].

MTI can also be used to assess global MS lesion burden by means of MTR histogram analysis [41]. This is a highly automated technique able to provide several metrics reflecting both macro- and microscopic MS pathology in the whole brain or in selected regions. MTR histogram measures can distinguish MS patients from healthy controls [25, 41, 42]. MS patients typically have lower average MTR, histogram peak height and position than normal subjects. However, MTR histogram parameters can be different in the various clinical forms of MS [42]. Patients with clinically isolated syndromes (CIS) suggestive of MS have MTR histogram-derived metrics similar to those from healthy controls, whereas PPMS patients have significantly lower histogram peak height with normal peak position and only slightly reduced average MTR. RRMS patients have lower average MTR and peak height than benign MS, whose histograms are similar to those of healthy subjects. Patients with SPMS had the lowest MTR histogram metrics. On the basis of these results, it can be concluded that MTR histogram-derived measures can provide insights into the pathogenesis of the different MS phenotypes. For instance, the reported findings suggest that, in PPMS, a subtle but widespread damage of the NAWM seems to be the major contributor to the neurological impairment. Other studies have found that MTR histogram metrics are also well correlated with the presence of neuropsychological impairment in MS patients [43, 44], and that MTR histogram parameters from the cerebellum and brainstem of MS patients are significantly associated with impairment in these functional systems [45].

Macroscopic lesions segmented on T2-weighted images can be superimposed onto the co-registered MTR maps and the areas corresponding to the segmented lesions can be nulled out, thus obtaining MTR maps of normal-appearing brain tissue (NABT). A recent study [46] using such an approach demonstrated that NABT-MTR histogram measures are different in the different MS clinical phenotypes and that changes in the NABT are only partially correlated with the extent of macroscopic lesions and the severity of intrinsic lesion damage, thus suggesting that NABT changes do not only reflect wallerian degeneration of axons traversing large focal abnormalities. Using a multivariate analysis of several MRI and MTI variables, Filippi et al. [47] found that average NABT-MTR was the only factor significantly associated with cognitive impairment in MS patients.

Recently, it has been shown that it is possible to acquire MT images of the cervical cord of good quality [48]. Using cervical cord MT histogram analysis, it has been reported that, in MS patients, MTR histogram measures correlate well with locomotor disability [49] and do not differ from those obtained in patients with Devic's neuromyelitis optica (DNO) [50].

MTI has also been used to assess the tissue damage within and outside T2-visible lesions of many WMD. MTR values for MS lesions visible on T2-weighted scans are significantly lower than those of lesions from elderly patients [51], or from patients with migraine [52], small-vessel disease [36], HIV encephalitis [53], CNS tuberculosis [54], systemic lupus erythematosus (SLE) [55, 56], or other systemic autoimmune diseases (including Wegener granulomatosis, Behçet disease, and APLAS) [56]. Moderately reduced MTR has also been found in white matter hyperintensities of patients with vascular dementia [57] and in the cortico-spinal tract of patients with amyotrophic lateral sclerosis [58]. Markedly decreased MTR values have been found in lesions from patients with progressive multifocal leukoencephalopathy (PML) [53], central pontine myelinolysis [59], or cerebral autosomal dominant arteriopathy with subcortical infarcts and leukoencephalopathy (CADASIL) [60]. Regardless of the average lesion MTR values found in these WMD, the lesions of MS tend to have a greater variability in their MTR values, possibly as a consequence of their temporal heterogeneity. MTR changes in the NAWM have been found in patients with neurological SLE [56], CADASIL [60], PML [53], HIV encephalitis [53] and head trauma [61], but not in the other WMD, including patients with DNO [50]. Although MTR changes in T2-visible lesions and NAWM are not disease specific, they may give important diagnostic information. For example, in patients with AIDS, MTI improves the differentiation between PML and HIV-associated white matter lesions [53, 62]. The absence of MTR changes in NAWM from patients with migraine and multiple T2 lesions reasonably excludes the presence of MS [52]. The absence of MTR changes in NAWM in patients with optic neuropathy and myelopathy increases the confidence in making a diagnosis of DNO [50].

Diffusion-Weighted Imaging

Diffusion is the random translational motion of molecules in a fluid system. In the brain, diffusion is influenced by the microstructural components of tissue, including cell membranes and organelles. The diffusion coefficient of biological tissues (which can be measured in vivo by MRI) is, therefore, lower than the diffusion coefficient in free water [63], and, for this reason, is named apparent diffusion coefficient (ADC). Pathological processes that modify tissue integrity, thus resulting in a loss of "restricting" barriers, can determine an increase of the ADC. Since some cellular structures are aligned on the scale of an image pixel, the measurement of diffusion is also dependent on the direction in which diffusion is measured. As a consequence, diffusion measurements can give information about the size, shape, and orientation of tissues [64]. A measure of diffusion that is independent of the orientation of structures is provided by the mean diffusivity, $\bar{D}$, the average of the ADCs measured in three orthogonal directions. A full characterization of diffusion can be obtained in terms of a tensor [65], a 3x3 matrix which accounts for the correlation existing between molecular displacement along orthogonal directions. From the tensor, it is possible to derive $\bar{D}$, equal to one-third of its trace, and some other dimensionless indexes of anisotropy. One of the most used is the fractional anisotropy (FA) [66].

DWI has proved to be of great clinical utility in the assessment of patients with cerebral ischemia. Using DWI, it is possible to identify the location and the extent of the ischemic event earlier and more precisely than using conventional scanning. ADC decreases within a few minutes after cessation of blood flow, while it appears to return to normal and, then, to overshoot after a few days [67-70]. The reduction of ADC soon after an ischemic event may be the result of water moving from the extracellular to the intracellular space, which is a more-restricted environment. Since the ADC reduction of the injured brain tissue is closely correlated with the temporal development of infarction and the degree of ischemic injury, the onset of the ischemic event can be estimated [71]. Experiments with reversible ischemic models have also shown that the ADC reduction during ischemia can be reversed after reperfusion. This suggests that DWI has the potential for identifying areas of compromised but recoverable tissue and for monitoring treatment efficacy [72].

The pathological elements of MS alter the permeability or geometry of structural barriers to water diffusion in the brain. The application of DWI techniques to MS is, therefore, appealing in the sense that they can provide a quantitative estimate of the degree of tissue damage and might increase the understanding of the mechanisms leading to irreversible disability. In experimental allergic encephalomyelitis, an animal model of MS, DWI signal intensity increased before any detectable change on T2-weighted scans [73] and increased ADC was seen in lesions [73], with a relatively preserved diffusion anisotropy in chronic compared with acute lesions [74]. The first report of water diffusion in MS showed that MS lesions had increased ADC values compared with NAWM [75]. The highest ADC were found in lesions less than 3 months old [75]. A subsequent study [76], with more-stable diffusion measurements, confirmed the preliminary results and demonstrated that NAWM of MS patients had higher ADC values than white matter from controls. However, these studies suffered from motion artefact, limited brain coverage, and the application of diffusion gradients in a single direction. Nevertheless, their results were confirmed by a later study [77], which used a volume-selective technique that allowed relatively rapid ADC measurements in three orthogonal directions without major motion artefact. This study [77] also detected similar ADC in lesions from SPMS and benign MS. A more-recent study [78] used a navigator echo strategy to correct for motion artefact in a spin-echo diffusion sequence and cover larger portions of the brain than previous studies [75-77]. Again, previous results were confirmed and a significantly increased $\bar{D}$ was found in T1-hypointense compared with T1-isointense lesions, and in non-enhancing compared with enhancing lesions [78].

Many of the problems of these studies [75-78] can be addressed by the use of echo-planar imaging (EPI), which is less prone to motion and permits greater brain coverage, with more diffusion gradient directions, in a given time. Recent studies [79-81] used such an approach and achieved the following results. $\bar{D}$ values of NAWM from MS patients are diffusely lower than the corresponding $\bar{D}$ values of white matter from controls; T2-visible lesions have lower $\bar{D}$ values than NAWM; hypointense T1 lesions have the lowest $\bar{D}$ values. Conflicting results have been obtained when comparing enhancing and non-enhancing lesions. One study [79] confirmed that enhancing lesions have higher $\bar{D}$ values and another [81], which assessed more patients, did not find any significant difference between the two lesion groups. FA has also been found to be reduced within and outside T2-visible lesions [79, 82]. Among lesions, FA was lower in enhancing than non-enhancing lesions [79]. All these data suggest a diffuse loss of structural barriers to water molecular motion in NAWM from MS patients. As expected, the loss of structural barriers is even greater in macroscopic lesions and its magnitude seems to be correlated with the intrinsic tissue damage. Since "inflammatory" changes and gliosis could potentially restrict water molecular motion, myelin and axonal loss are the most-likely contributors to the increased $\bar{D}$ and decreased FA in MS NAWM and lesions. The correlation between the average $\bar{D}$ values in the lesions and NAWM has been investigated in one study and found not to be significant [80]. This again suggests that subtle NAWM changes are not merely the result of wallerian degeneration of axons traversing larger lesions. Recent work detected $\bar{D}$ and MTR changes in the gray matter of MS patients [83].

As for MT, the analysis of diffusion changes can also be performed on a more-global basis using $\bar{D}$ histograms [80]. MS patients have significantly higher average $\bar{D}$ and lower histogram peak height than normals. Histogram broadening, and the consequent decrease of peak height, shows that fewer pixels in patients' brain have normal $\bar{D}$ values. The magnitude of the correlation between MTR and $\bar{D}$ has also been investigated [80]. In MS lesions, a strong inverse correlation between average MTR and $\bar{D}$ was found [80]. However, this correlation was not found when considering NAWM-ROI and the brain by means of histograms [80]. The lack of correlation between MTR and $\bar{D}$ in the brain tissue might be the result of the complex relationship between destructive and reparative mechanisms occurring in the NAWM and their variable effects on MTR and $\bar{D}$ values.

Although challenging, diffusion has also been studied in the optic nerve of MS patients [84]. Increased ADC has been found in the affected optic nerves [84].

While DWI has been extensively used to investigate acute stroke and is starting to be used to assess tissue damage in MS, its application in other WMD is still marginal. A study of diffusion characteristics in patients affected by leukoaraiosis [85] demonstrated an increased $\bar{D}$ and reduced FA in the damaged tissue. An elevation in the $\bar{D}$ and a reduction in the FA has also been shown in the posterior limb of the internal capsule in patients with ALS [86].

Conclusions

Conventional MRI has markedly increased our ability to detect the macroscopic abnormalities of the brain and spinal cord associated with WMD. New quantitative MR approaches with increased sensitivity to subtle NAWM changes and increased specificity to the heterogeneous pathological substrates of WMD lesions may provide information complementary to conventional MRI. MTI and DWI have the potential to provide relevant information on the structural changes occurring within and outside T2-visible lesions. MRS could add information on the biochemical nature of such changes. Their extensive application should improve the understanding of the mechanisms leading to irreversible disability and help in the diagnostic work-up of many WMD, as is already the case for MS. Multiparametric MRI studies are now warranted to better define the nature of the pathological damage in individual pathological conditions, and, hopefully, to evaluate the efficacy of experimental treatment in preventing the formation of "disabling" lesions.

References

1. Davie CA, Hawkins CP, Barker GJ et al (1994) Serial proton magnetic resonance spectroscopy in acute multiple sclerosis lesions. Brain 117:49-58
2. De Stefano N, Matthews PM, Antel JP et al (1995) Chemical pathology of acute demyelinating lesions and its correlation with disability. Ann Neurol 38:901-909
3. Narayana PA, Doyle TJ, Lai D, Wolinsky JS (1998) Serial proton magnetic resonance spectroscopic imaging, contrast- enhanced magnetic resonance imaging, and quantitative lesion volumetry in multiple sclerosis. Ann Neurol 43:56-71
4. Arnold DL, Matthews PM, Francis GS et al (1992) Proton magnetic resonance spectroscopic imaging for metabolic characterization of demyelinating plaques. Ann Neurol 31:235-241
5. De Stefano N, Matthews PM, Arnold DL (1995) Reversible decreases in N-acetylaspartate after acute brain injury. Magn Reson Med 34:721-727
6. Falini A, Calabrese G, Filippi M et al (1998) Benign versus secondary progressive multiple sclerosis: the potential role of 1H MR spectroscopy in defining the nature of disability. AJNR Am J Neuroradiol 19:223-229
7. Arnold DL, Riess GT, Matthews PM et al (1994) Use of proton magnetic resonance spectroscopy for monitoring disease progression in multiple sclerosis. Ann Neurol 36:76-82

8. Davie CA, Barker GJ, Webb S et al (1995) Persistent functional deficit in multiple sclerosis and autosomal dominant cerebellar ataxia is associated with axon loss. Brain 118:1583-1592

9. Matthews PM, Pioro E, Narayanan S et al (1996) Assessment of lesion pathology in multiple sclerosis using quantitative MRI morphometry and magnetic resonance spectroscopy. Brain 119:715-722

10. De Stefano N, Matthews PM, Fu L et al (1998) Axonal damage correlates with disability in patients with relapsing- remitting multiple sclerosis. Results of a longitudinal magnetic resonance spectroscopy study. Brain 121:1469-1477

11. Filippi M, Tortorella C, Bozzali M (1999) Normal-appearing white matter changes in multiple sclerosis: the contribution of magnetic resonance techniques. Mult Scler 5:273-282

12. De Stefano N, Narayanan S, Matthews PM et al (1999) In vivo evidence for axonal dysfunction remote from focal cerebral demyelination of the type seen in multiple sclerosis. Brain 122:1933-1939

13. Davie CA, Barker GJ, Thompson AJ et al (1997) 1H magnetic resonance spectroscopy of chronic cerebral white matter lesions and normal appearing white matter in multiple sclerosis. J Neurol Neurosurg Psychiatry 63:736-742

14. Fu L, Matthews PM, De Stefano N et al (1998) Imaging of axonal damage of normal appearing white matter in multiple sclerosis. Brain 121:103-113

15. De Stefano N, Federico A, Arnold DL (1997) Proton magnetic resonance spectroscopy in brain white matter disorders. Ital J Neurol Sci 18: 331-339

16. Austin SJ, Connelly A, Gadian DG et al (1991) Localized 1H NMR spectroscopy in Canavan's disease: a report of two cases. Magn Reson Med 19:439-445

17. van der Knaap MS, Wevers RA, Struys EA et al (1995) Leukoencephalopathy with swelling and a discrepantly mild clinical course in eight children. Ann Neurol 37:324-334

18. Ross BD, Bluml S, Cowan R et al (1997) In vivo magnetic resonance spectroscopy of human brain: the biophysical basis of dementia. Biophys Chem 68:161-172

19. Bruhn H, Kruse B, Korenke GC et al (1992) Proton NMR spectroscopy of cerebral metabolic alterations in infantile peroxisomal disorders. J Comput Assist Tomogr 16:335-344

20. Johannik K, Van Hecke P, Francois B et al (1994) Localized brain proton NMR spectroscopy in young adult phenylketonuria patients. Magn Reson Med 31:53-57

21. Tzika AA, Ball WS Jr, Vigneron DB et al (1993) Childhood adrenoleukodystrophy: assessment with proton MR spectroscopy. Radiology 189:467-480

22. Kruse B, Hanefeld F, Christen HJ et al (1993) Alterations of brain metabolites in metachromatic leukodystrophy as detected by localized proton magnetic resonance spectroscopy in vivo. J Neurol 241:68-74

23. van der Knaap MS, van der Grond J, Luyten PR et al (1992) ^{1}H and ^{31}P magnetic resonance spectroscopy of the brain in degenerative cerebral disorders. Ann Neurol 31:202-211

24. Kruse B, Barker PB, van Zijl PC et al (1994) Multislice proton magnetic resonance spectroscopic imaging in X- linked adrenoleukodystrophy. Ann Neurol 36:595-608

25. Filippi M, Grossman RI, Comi G (eds) (1999) Magnetization transfer in multiple sclerosis. Neurology 53 [Suppl 3]

26. van Waesberghe JH, Kamphorst W, De Groot CJ et al (1999) Axonal loss in multiple sclerosis lesions: magnetic resonance imaging insights into substrates of disability. Ann Neurol 46:747-754

27. Dousset V, Dousset V, Grossman RI, Ramer KN et al (1992) Experimental allergic encephalomyelitis and multiple sclerosis: lesion characterization with magnetization transfer imaging. Radiology 182:483-491

28. Lai HM, Davie CA, Gass A et al (1997) Serial magnetization transfer ratios in gadolinium-enhancing lesions in multiple sclerosis. J Neurol 244:308-311

29. Campi A, Filippi M, Comi G et al (1996) Magnetization transfer ratios of contrast-enhancing and nonenhancing lesions in multiple sclerosis. Neuroradiology 38:115-119

30. Hiehle JF, Grossman RI, Ramer NK et al (1995) Magnetization transfer effects in MR-detected multiple sclerosis lesions: comparison with gadolinium-enhanced spin-echo images and non-enhanced T1-weighted images. AJNR Am J Neuroradiol 16:69-77

31. Petrella JR, Grossman RI, McGowan JC et al (1996) Multiple sclerosis lesions: relationship between MR enhancement pattern and magnetization transfer effect. AJNR Am J Neuroradiol 17:1041-1049

32. Filippi M, Rocca MA, Rizzo G et al (1998) Magnetization transfer ratios in MS lesions enhancing after different doses of gadolinium. Neurology 50:1289-1293

33. Filippi M, Rocca MA, Comi G (1998) Magnetization transfer ratios of multiple sclerosis lesions with variable durations of enhancement. J Neurol Sci 159:162-165

34. Rocca MA, Mastronardo G, Rodegher M et al (1999) Long term changes of MT-derived measures from patients with relapsing-remitting and secondary-progressive multiple sclerosis. AJNR Am J Neuroadiol 20:821-827

35. Filippi M, Rocca MA, Martino G et al (1998) Magnetization transfer changes in the normal appearing white matter precede the appearance of enhancing lesions in patients with multiple sclerosis. Ann Neurol 43:809-814

36. Gass A, Barker GJ, Kidd D et al (1994) Correlation of magnetization transfer ratio with disability in multiple sclerosis. Ann Neurol 36:62-67

37. van Waesberghe JHTM, van Walderveen MA, Castelijns JA et al (1998) Patterns of lesion development in multiple sclerosis: longitudinal observations with T1-weighted spin-echo and magnetization MR. AJNR Am J Neuroradiol 19:675-683

38. Filippi M, Campi A, Dousset V et al (1995) A magnetization transfer imaging study of normal-appearing white matter in multiuple sclerosis. Neurology 45:478-482

39. Loevner LA, Grossman RI, Cohen JA et al (1995) Microscopic disease in normal-appearing white matter on conventional MR imaging in patients with multiple sclerosis: assessment with magnetization-transfer measurements. Radiology 196:511-515

40. Filippi M, Rocca MA, Minicucci L et al (1999) Magnetization transfer imaging of patients with definite MS and negative conventional MRI. Neurology 52:845-848

41. van Buchem MA, McGowan JC, Kolson DL et al (1996) Quantitative volumetric magnetization transfer analysis in multiple sclerosis: estimation of macroscopic and microscopic disease burden. Magn Reson Med 36:632-636

42. Filippi M, Iannucci G, Tortorella C et al (1999) Comparison of MS clinical phenotypes using conventional and magnetization transfer MRI. Neurology 52:588-594

43. Rovaris M, Filippi M, Falautano M et al (1998) Relation between MR abnormalities and patterns of cognitive impairment in multiple sclerosis. Neurology 50:1601-1608

44. van Buchem MA, Grossman RI, Armstrong C et al (1998) Correlation of volumetric magnetization transfer imaging with clinical data in MS. Neurology 50:1609-1617

45. Iannucci G, Minicucci L, Rodegher M et al (1999) Correlations between clinical and MRI involvement in multiple sclerosis: assessment using T1, T2 and MT histograms. J Neurol Sci 171:121-129

46. Tortorella C, Viti B, Bozzali M et al (2000) A magnetization transfer histogram study of normal appearing brain tissue in multiple sclerosis. Neurology 54:186-193

47. Filippi M, Tortorella C, Rovaris M et al (2000) Changes in the normal appearing brain tissue and cognitive impairment in multiple sclerosis. J Neurol Neurosurg Psychiatry 68:157-161

48. Bozzali M, Rocca MA, Iannucci G et al (1999) Magnetization transfer histogram analysis of the cervical cord in patients wth multiple sclerosis. AJNR Am J Neuroradiol 20:1803-1808

49. Filippi M, Bozzali M, Horsfield MA et al (2000) A conventional and magnetization transfer MRI study of the cervical cord in patients with multiple sclerosis. Neurology 54:207-213

50. Filippi M, Rocca MA, Moiola L et al (1999) MRI and MTI changes in the brain and cervical cord from patients with Devic's neuromyelitis optica. Neurology 53:1705-1710

51. Wong KT, Grossman RI, Boorstein JM et al (1995) Magnetization transfer imaging of periventricular hyperintense white matter in the elderly. AJNR Am J Neuroadiol 16:253-258

52. Rocca MA, Colombo B, Pratesi A et al (2000) A magnetization transfer imaging study of the brain in patients with migraine. Neurology 54:507-509

53. Dousset V, Armand JP, Lacoste D et al (1997) Magnetization transfer study of HIV encephalitis and progressive multifocal leukoencephalopathy. AJNR Am J Neuroradiol 18:859-901

54. Gupta RK, Kathuria KM, Pradhan S (1999) Magnetization transfer MR imaging in CNS tubercolosis. AJNR Am J Neuroradiol 20:867-875

55. Campi A, Filippi M, Gerevini S et al (1996) Multiple white matter lesions of the brain. Magnetization transfer ratios in systemic lupus erythematosus and multiple sclerosis. Int J Neuroradiol 2:134-140

56. Rovaris M, Viti B, Ciboddo G et al (1999) Brain involvement in systemic immune-mediated diseases: a magnetic resonance and magnetization transfer imaging study. J Neurol Neurosurg Psychiatry 68:170-177

57. Tanabe JL, Ezekiel F, Jagust WJ et al (1999) Magnetization transfer ratio of white matter hyperintensities in subcortical ischemic vascular dementia. AJNR Am J Neuroradiol 20:839-844

58. Kato Y, Matsumura K, Kinosada Y et al (1997) Detection of pyramidal tract lesions in amyotrophic lateral sclerosis with magnetization-transfer measurements. AJNR Am J Neuroradiol 18:1541-1547

59. Silver NC, Barker GJ, MacManus DG et al (1996) Decreased magnetization transfer ratio due to demyelination: a case of central pontine myelinolysis. J Neurol Neurosurg Psychiatry 61:208-209

60. Iannucci G, Dichgans M, Rovaris M et al (2000) Correlations between clinical findings and magnetization transfer imaging metrics of tissue damage in individuals with cerebral autosomal dominant arteriopathy with subcortical infarcts and leukoencephalopathy. Stroke 32:643-648

61. Bagley LJ, Grossman RI, Galetta SL et al (1999) Characterization of white matter lesions in multiple sclerosis and traumatic brain injury as revealed by magnetization transfer contour plots. AJNR Am J Neuroradiol 20:977-981

62. Ernst T, Chang L, Witt M et al (1999) Progressive multifocal leukoencephalopathy and human immunodeficiency virus-associated white matter lesions in AIDS: magnetization transfer MR imaging. Radiology 210:539-543

63. Woessner DE (1963) NMR spin-echo self-diffusion measurement on fluids undergoing restricted diffusion. J Phys Chem 67:1365-1367

64. Le Bihan D, Turner R, Pekar J, Moonen CTW (1991) Diffusion and perfusion imaging by gradient sensitization: design, startegy and significance. J Magn Reson Imaging 1:7-8

65. Basser PJ, Mattiello J, LeBihan D (1994) MR diffusion tensor spectroscopy and imaging. Biophys J 66:259-267

66. Pierpaoli C, Basser PJ (1996) Toward a quantitative assessment of diffusion anisotropy. Magn Reson Med 36:893-906

67. Moseley ME, Kucharczyk J, Mintorovitch J et al (1990) Diffusion-weighted MR imaging of acute stroke: correlation with T2-weighted and magnetic susceptibility enhanced MR imaging in cats. AJNR Am J Neuroradiol 14:423-429

68. Moseley ME, Cohen Y, Mintorovitch J et al (1990) Early detection of regional cerebral ischemia in cats: comparison of diffusion- and T2 weighted MRI and spectroscopy. Magn Reson Med 14:330-346

69. Warach S, Chien D, Li W et al (1992) Fast magnetic resonance diffusion-weighted imaging of acute human stroke. Neurology 42:1717-1723

70. Lutsep HL, Albers GW, DeCrespigny A et al (1997) Clinical utility of diffusion-weighted magnetic resonance imaging in the assessment of ischaemic stroke. Ann Neurol 41:574-580

71. Schlaug G, Siewert B, Benfield A et al (1997) Time course of the apparent diffusion coefficient (ADC) abnormality in human stroke. Neurology 49:113-119

72. Minematsu K, Li L, Sotak CH et al (1992) Reversible focal ischemic injury demonstrated by diffusion-weighted magnetic resonance imaging in rats. Stroke 23:1304-1311

73. Heide AC, Richards TL, Alvord EC Jr et al (1993) Diffusion imaging of experimental allergic encephalomyelitis. Magn Reson Med 4:478-484

74. Verhoye MR, Gravenmade EJ, Raman ER et al (1996) In vivo noninvasive determination of abnormal water diffusion in the rat brain studied in an animal model for multiple sclerosis by diffusion-weighted NMR imaging. Magn Reson Imaging 14:521-532

75. Larsson HBW, Thomsen C, Frederiksen J et al (1992) In vivo magnetic resonance diffusion measurement in the brain of patients with multiple sclerosis. Magn Reson Imaging 10:7-12

76. Christiansen P, Gideon P, Thomsen C et al (1993) Increased water self-diffusion in chronic plaques and in apparently normal white matter in patients with multiple sclerosis. Acta Neurol Scand 87:195-199

77. Horsfield MA, Lai M, Webb SL et al (1996) Apparent diffusion coefficient in benign and in secondary progressive multiple sclerosis by nuclear magnetic resonance. Magn Reson Med 36:393-400

78. Droogan AG, Clark CA, Werring DJ et al (1999) Comparison of multiple sclerosis clinical subgroups using navigated spin echo diffusion-weighted imaging. Magn Reson Imaging 17:653-661

79. Werring DJ, Clark CA, Barker GJ et al (1999) Diffusion tensor imaging of lesions and normal-appearing white matter in multiple sclerosis. Neurology 52:1626-1632

80. Cercignani M, Iannucci G, Rocca MA et al (2000) Pathologic damage in MS assessed by diffusion-weighted and magnetization transfer MRI. Neurology 54:1139-1144

81. Filippi M, Iannucci G, Cercignani M et al (2000) A quantitative study of water diffusion in MS lesions and NAWM using echo-planar imaging. Arch Neurol 57:1017-1021

82. Filippi M, Cercignani M, Inglese M et al (2001) Diffusion tensor magnetic resonance imaging in multiple sclerosis. Neurology 56:304-311

83. Cercignani M, Bozzali M, Iannucci G et al (2001) Magnetisation transfer ratio and mean diffusivity of normal-appearing white and gray matter from patients with multiple sclerosis. J Neurol Neurosurg Psychiatry 70:311-317

84. Iwasawa T, Matoba H, Ogi A et al (1997) Diffusion-weighted imaging of the human optic nerve: a new approach to evaluate optic neuritis in multiple sclerosis. Magn Reson Med 38:484-491

85. Jones DK, Lythgoe D, Horsfield MA et al (1999) Characterization of white matter damage in ischaemic leukoaraiosis with diffusion tensor MRI. Stroke 30:393-397

86. Ellis CM, Simmons A, Jones DK et al (1999) Diffusion tensor MRI assesses corticospinal tract damage in ALS. Neurology 53:1051-1058

Monounsaturated Fatty Acids and Neuroprotection. The Results of a Study of Cognitive Decline in Old Age. Is There a Case for this Treatment in Multiple Sclerosis?

A. Capurso, F. Panza, V. Solfrizzi, C. Capurso, A. D'Introno, S. Capurso, A.M. Colacicco

Introduction

Different diagnostic criteria have been proposed to distinguish individuals with mild cognitive disorders associated with aging. One of the best established of these classifications is age-associated memory impairment (AAMI) [1], but it is generally non-progressive and is thus more likely to be a phenomenon of normal aging [2, 3]. The terms "age-related cognitive decline" (ARCD) and "aging-associated cognitive decline" have been proposed recently [4, 5] to indicate an objective decline in cognitive functioning associated with the aging process but within normal limits given the person's age. Whether ARCD is an expression of a normal aging process, represents a distinct clinical entity, or is a continuum with dementia is still difficult to establish [2, 6]. Recent results from longitudinal studies suggest that the subgroup at high risk for developing dementia may be identified by using a more-detailed procedure for the assessment of cognitive decline than those listed in the AAMI criteria. A high incidence (45%) of dementia was found in individuals aged >75 years who were diagnosed as having "minimal dementia" by the CAMDEX interview [7]. Furthermore, in another study 48% of patients with isolated memory loss of unknown cause developed dementia within 3.7 years [8].

The causes of ARCD are unknown, but some studies have suggested that it may be prevented [9]. Cardiovascular and other chronic diseases [10, 11], hypertension [12], diabetes mellitus [13], depression [14], and a low level of physical activity have been identified as risk factors for ARCD [15]. In contrast, a high socioeconomic status, a flexible personality in middle age, and maintenance of vision and hearing have been identified as factors protective against ARCD [16].

The role of the diet in ARCD has not been extensively investigated. Deficiencies of micronutrients (B_1, B_2, B_6, B_{12}, C vitamins, and folate) have been frequently described in elderly people and significantly associated with cognitive impairment [17, 18]. However, very few data are available on the role of macronutrient intake in ARCD [19]. In a recent study, we investigated the relationships between dietary macronutrient intakes and age-related changes in cognitive functions [20-22]. The subjects of this study take part in a larger study, the "Italian Longitudinal Study on Aging" (ILSA), promoted by the Italian National Research Council (CNR) Targeted Project on Aging [23]. This was an Italian multicenter, population-based cohort study, with both survey and prospective components, designed to evaluate age-related diseases, as well as physiological and functional changes of cardiovascular, endocrine, metabolic, and nervous systems in the aging process. A sample of 5,632 subjects aged 65-84 years, living at home or institutionalized, was randomly selected from the electoral rolls of eight municipalities [Genoa, Segrate (Milan), Selvazzano-Rubano (Padua), Impruneta (Florence), Fermo (Ascoli-Piceno), Naples, Casamassima (Bari), and Catania] after stratification for age and gender. The data of this study have been obtained during the prevalence survey study carried out in Casamassima (Bari, Southern Italy) between March 1992 and June 1993 (prevalence day 1 March, 1992). Of 704 randomized elderly subjects, 404 (57.4%) agreed to participate, and the study population consisted of 278 non-demented elderly subjects, living at home, who performed both the neuropsychological evaluation and the dietary assessment. Criteria for study entry included no known diagnoses of brain tumor, cerebrovascular malformations, psychosis, epilepsy, multiple sclerosis (MS), stage III syphilis, Parkinson's disease, stroke (atherothrombotic, hemorrhagic brain infarction, or transient ischemic attack), and dementia. Furthermore, no severe functional limitations and no treatment with any drug that could interfere with the parameters of the study protocol were allowed.

Mini Mental State Examination (MMSE) was used to evaluate global cognitive functions (orientation in space and time, concentration and attention span, immediate and delayed verbal memory, constructive praxis, and language) [24]. Episodic memory was explored with Babcock Story Recall Test (BSRT) (score ranging from 0 to 16) [25, 26]. This test measures, with a 21-unit story, immediate and delayed recall, and their sum. Selective attention was assessed by Digit Cancellation Test (DCT) (score ranging from 0 to 60) [25]. The food intake was assessed with a 77-item semi-quantitative food frequency questionnaire, which had been previously validated. Dietary variables estimated were: energy, total lipids, saturated fatty acids (SFA), monounsaturated fatty acids (MUFA), polyunsaturated fatty acids (PUFA), carbohydrates, proteins, alcohol, total, insoluble, and soluble fibers, cellulose, and non-cellulosic polysaccharides. Height and weight were measured for each participant: vertical stature was measured to the nearest 0.01 m with a stadiometer, weight was measured to the nearest 0.1 kg with an electronic balance, and body mass index (BMI) ($= kg/m^2$) was calculated.

Spearman's non-parametric correlation was performed to evaluate the relationships between cognitive and nutritional variables. Subsequently, a multivariate logistic regression model was used to evaluate any significant change in odds ratios of cognitive impairment for macronutrient intakes (Table 1). These relationships were controlled for covariates that could be effective modifiers, and/or confounders, such as age, gender, education, and BMI.

Table 1. Change in odds ratio of cognitive decline, Mini Mental State Examination <24 (MMSE) for monounsaturated acid (MUFA) energy intake controlling for education and age, the Italian Longitudinal Study on Aging-Casamassima, First prevalence Survey, 1992-1993 (modified from [21]) (*CI* confidence interval)

MUFA intake (kJ/day)	MUFA adjusting for education		MUFA adjusting for education and age	
	Odds ratio	95% CI	Odds ratio	95% CI
≤800	33	8.2 - 133	37.5	9 - 156
801-1200	14.9	6.2 - 35.8	16.9	6.7 - 42.7
1201-1600	6.7	3.7 - 12	7.6	3.9 - 14.6
1601-2000	3	1.3 - 6.7	3.4	1.4 - 8
2001-2400	1.3	0.4 - 4.9	1.5	0.4 - 5.8
2401-2800	0.6	0.1 - 4.5	0.69	0.1 - 4.5

MUFA and ARCD

In this study, neuropsychological test scores and macronutrient intakes appeared mutually independent, except for MUFA intakes, which were significantly associated with an improvement in odds ratio of global cognitive functions and selective attention. Furthermore, the effect of education on the odds of having cognitive impairment decreases exponentially with MUFA energy intake. These findings appear to be consistent with other studies; they indicate an association between dietary intake and cognitive function. In a recent longitudinal study of a well-nourished and cognitively unimpaired elderly community residents, a significant association between protein intake and cognitive performance was found [27]. In another study, a significant association between functional variables (i.e., activities of daily living) and alcohol intake was found, likely in relation to the better health status of moderate alcohol consumers [28]. Finally, in a recent study, non-institutionalized elderly subjects with the best performance in cognitive tests had lower intake of MUFAs, SFAs, and cholesterol, and higher intakes of total food, fruit, carbohydrate, thiamine, folate, and vitamin C [29]. These apparently conflicting results could be partially due to some methodological differences in food frequency questionnaires and selection of participants, which was not performed randomly, but within three elderly persons' clubs.

Due to the dietary pattern of our population, the typical Mediterranean diet, and to the rural setting of the study (Casamassima), the mean consumption of olive oil was particularly high: 46 g/day (12.6 range 113.1 g/day). MUFA energy intake was 17.6%, 85% of which was derived from olive oil. The positive effect of dietary habits on cognitive functioning of healthy elderly subjects could be due in part to the antioxidant components of olive oil, i.e., tocopherols and polyphenols. Some pathological conditions, which can be triggered by an uncontrolled production of free radicals, could probably be prevented or retarded with high intakes of dietary antioxidants (i.e., vitamins A, E, C, and carotenes). These might yield beneficial effects on frontal/subcortical brain systems, with enhancement of cognitive functions (increased performance on memory tasks) [30-32]. However, the antioxidant effect of dietary macronutrients could not exert under every circumstance a protective effect on age-related changes in cognitive functions. In a Japanese study [16], a high dietary intake of antioxidant compounds was significantly associated with Alzheimer's disease and ARCD.

High MUFA intake *per se* could suggest preservation of cognitive functions in healthy elderly people. This effect could be related to the role of fatty acids in maintaining the structural integrity of neuronal membranes. A recent study on fatty acid composition of neuronal membranes demonstrated an increase in MUFA content and a decrease in PUFA content with advancing age [33]. It seems that during the aging process there is an increasing demand for unsaturated fatty acids. In lymphocytic and macrophage-like cells, an increase of Δ^9 desaturase activity, which converts stearic acid to oleic acid and increases the degree of differentiation of cells, has been observed [34]. These findings are consistent with another recent study in which high PUFA intake was positively associated with cognitive impairment, while high fish consumption tended to be inversely associated with cognitive impairment [35].

Supplementation of PUFA in MS

Our data have demonstrated that high intakes of MUFA in elderly people are associated with better performances in cognitive function tests, so we postulated that ARCD in the elderly should be slowed down by high intakes of unsaturated fatty acids, particularly monounsaturated oleic acid. Whether MUFA are protective in other neuropathological contexts needs to be demonstrated.

MS is a major demyelinating disease characterized by destruction of myelin and marked alteration of myelin lipids. The pathogenesis of MS is largely unknown. However, diet, particularly dietary fatty acids, have been demonstrated to influence the course of MS. In 1950, Swank [36] suggested that consumption of saturated animal fat was directly related to the incidence of MS. Furthermore, the incidence of MS was higher in the inland dairy eating populations of Norway than in the coastal fish-eating populations [37]. Statistical analysis of similar data from many geographic areas supported these findings [38, 39].

The myelin sheath of nerves is composed predominantly of lipids, and a lipid imbalance involving the essential fatty acids could affect cell fluidity, myelination, and synthesis of prostaglandins or other immunoregulatory compounds [40]. It was also suggested that animal fats could result in platelet aggregation with subsequent small vessel occlusion, which might cause perivascular plaques [37]. Finally, the effects of dietary fats could be related to the fact that fatty acid components of brain phospholipids can be extensively modulated by dietary lipids

[41]. In particular, the PUFA content of neuronal cell membrane can be extensively changed by diet, so modifying the membrane fluidity and functions [42]. Furthermore, relative deficiencies in PUFA have been found in the brain and serum of MS patients [40]. A diet low in SFA and high in unsaturated fatty acids, with a supplement of fish oil, has been associated with decreased neurological disability in MS patients [37, 43]. Although this study was uncontrolled, it suggested that SFA are associated with clinical worsening, while unsaturated fatty acids are associated with clinical improvement of MS.

A double-blind trial, supplementing with linoleic acid a group of 87 MS patients who were not in relapse and with a disability score between 0 and 6 (according the Kurtzke Disability Scale) found no statistically significant differences after 28 months in the disability scale or in the relapse rate between the groups treated with linoleic acid and with placebo [44]. In contrast, there was a difference regarding severity and frequency of clinical relapses, which were greater for the patients who took the placebo. Subsequent studies on the therapeutic use of PUFA in MS have not always shown positive effects on the course of disease. This can be attributed mostly to the different criteria of patient selection (some with the remitting form of the disease, others with the progressive form) and to the different disability rating of patients at the beginning of the study [45, 46]. The studies were not long enough to show real modifications in the clinical course. However, variations in biochemical or immunological indicators of disease activity might show earlier modifications of the disease course. The n-3 and n-6 PUFA series could have different effects at the membrane level, on platelet activity and immune function, because they are precursors of prostaglandin classes of different and sometimes antagonistic activity [47].

The geographic pattern of MS has attracted considerable attention in recent decades, and it has been hypothesized and substantiated that the prevalence of MS increases with increasing distance from the equator, both north and south [48]. In a recent study, a significant, positive, and independent correlation of MS mortality with SFA, animal fat, animal minus fish fat, and latitude was found [49]. These results suggested that dietary fat could be involved in the incidence of or mortality from MS, and that both nutritional factors and latitude seem to be independently related to MS mortality.

Relationship of Dietary Fatty Acids and Immune-Mediated Inflammatory Mechanisms in MS

MS appears to be related to immune-mediated inflammatory mechanisms, initiated by CD40-CD40L interaction. CD40 is a phosphorylated 49-kDa glycoprotein expressed on a variety of cells, including B and T lymphocytes, monocytic lineage cells (monocytes, macrophages, and microglial cells), endothelial cells and others, that shares significant homology with the receptors for tumor necrosis factor -α (TNF-α), and is designated as a member of the nerve growth factor receptor superfamily [50]. CD40L is a 30 to 33-kDa cell surface glycoprotein belonging to the TNF family of cytokines. The legation of CD40L secreted by activated T cells to CD40 surface glycoprotein initiates immune-mediated inflammatory mechanisms. Activated T-helper cells expressing CD40L surface protein have been demonstrated in MS patient brain sections and not in normal controls. In experimentally induced allergic encephalo-myelitis in mice, the onset of illness was completely prevented by treatment with anti-CD40L monoclonal antibody, and the administration of monoclonal antibody after disease onset led to dramatic disease reduction [51]. The presence of T-helper cells expressing CD40L in brain tissue of MS patients suggests that blocking or modulation of CD40-CD40L-mediated cellular interaction may be a method for treating active MS.

The relationship of dietary components with inflammatory mechanisms could be due to the modulating effect of dietary fatty acids on the immune-mediated inflammatory process. Nutrition has been demonstrated to play an important role in modulation of an animal's immune system. Important correlations have been found between deficiencies of nutrients (protein, energy intake, fat-soluble vitamin A, D and E, B complex vitamins, vitamin C, and the minerals selenium, iron, zinc, and copper) and immune dysfunction [52]. In this context, some nutrients may influence the production and activity of pro-inflammatory cytokines. Lipids, in particular, have been demonstrated to have a large potential for modulating cytokine biology. MUFA have been demonstrated to decrease tissue responsiveness to cytokines; n-6 PUFA enhance interleukin (IL)-1 production, while n-3 PUFA have the opposite effect. In particular, IL-1 and IL-6 production is positively related to dietary intake of linoleic acid; also leukotriene B_4 production is positively related to dietary linoleic acid intake [53].

High dietary MUFA intake in middle-aged males has been demonstrated to decrease significantly the expression of intercellular adhesion molecule-1 (ICAM1) by peripheral blood mononuclear cells [54]. MUFA and dietary olive oil have also been found to reduce by 40% vascular cell adhesion molecule-1 (VCAM1) expression by endothelial cells, so reducing the potential recruitment of mononuclear inflammatory cells [55-57].

The observed effects could be related to the capacity of alimentary fats to alter the biological membrane phospholipid composition. The cell membrane PUFA content influences membrane functions, and consequently the activity of membrane-associated functional proteins (transporters, receptors, enzymes) and the production of signaling molecules from oxygenated linoleic and α-linolenic acid derivatives [42]. Consequently, the binding of cytokines to receptors and the G-protein activity could also be modified.

ApoE Genotype and MS

The presence of the apolipoprotein E (apoE) ε4 appears to play an important role in the onset and progression of MS, although it is not associated with a higher risk of developing the disease itself [58]. ApoE is the only serum apolipoprotein present in the extravascular fluid of the brain [59]. It is contained in HDL1-like particles, is the major lipid carrier protein in the brain, and plays an important role in lipid transport in the central nervous system (CNS) [60]. A tandem dimer repeat peptide of apoE induces neuronal endocytosis via a receptor-associated protein-sensitive pathway [61]. ApoE is the ligand of lipoproteins to the main lipoprotein receptor in nervous system, the LRP receptor (LDL-receptor related protein) [62, 63]. This receptor, which is a member of the LDL receptor family, is also expressed in a wide set of cells including hepatocytes, macrophages, smooth muscle cells, and neurons of the CNS [63]. The most-relevant function of LRP is lipoprotein endocytosis, but it also helps in regulating urokinase receptor expression on the cell surface, and helps the binding of α_2-macroglobulin-proteinase complexes, the clearance of these complexes and of the cytokines associated with complexes [64]. ApoE expression is increased in regenerating neural tissue. ApoE ε4 allele is associated with impaired neuronal repair. Since repair is essential to restore the CNS function following MS relapses, the apoE genotype modulates the clinical progression of the disease. The estimated frequency of ε4 in normal, middle-aged populations ranges from 0.14 to 0.27 in northern regions of Europe and from 0.10 to 0.12 in southern countries [65, 66]. In our recent study, the apoE allele frequencies observed in late-onset Alzheimer's disease (LOAD) patients, healthy centenarians, and middle-aged subjects are consistent with similar data of other Italian studies [64], but differ from those of other European populations, particularly for the ε4 allele frequency, which appears to be underexpressed in our sample [66]. Our study provides a novel finding that the apoE ε4 allele frequency decreases according to a geographic trend from northern to southern Europe in two highly selected populations, i.e., LOAD patients and centenarians. Also the MS mortality has a north to south decreasing trend in Europe, while the unsaturated/saturated fatty acid ratio has an opposite trend [49], suggesting that environmental and genetic factors might synergistically contribute to the decreased MS mortality in southern European regions.

In conclusion, dietary unsaturated fatty acids appear to slow the decline of cognitive functions in the elderly. Whether unsaturated fatty acids could exert beneficial effects in demyelinating illness, i.e., MS, cannot be excluded. We must consider that in our study only very high intakes of MUFA , i.e., 2,400-2,800 kJ/day, corresponding to about 80 g/day of MUFA and 110 g/die of olive oil, were associated with preservation of cognitive functions. Furthermore, the daily intake of extra-virgin olive oil as the only alimentary fat also included the anti oxidants naturally occurring in olive oil, i.e., tocopherol and polyphenols (25 mg/dl and 30-90 mg/dl, respectively). The concomitant intake of enough antioxidants to protect unsaturated fatty acids from oxidation could have had a role in the protective effects of olive oil. Moreover, unsaturated fatty acids modify membrane fluidity, and consequently the activity of membrane functions such as enzymes, receptors, and ion channels. Finally, MUFA have been demonstrated to influence tissue inflammatory mechanisms, decreasing tissue responsiveness to inflammatory cytokines and reducing the expression of the adhesion molecules VCAM1 and ICAM1 from mononuclear and endothelial cells, respectively.

Acknowledgements. The authors thank Dr. Giovanni Castellaneta for skillful assistance. This study was supported by the Italian Longitudinal Study on Aging (ILSA) (Italian National Research Council (CNR) Targeted Project on Aging grants 9400419PF40 and 95973PF40), by Targeted Project on Mediterranean Diet (Italian National Research Council – CNR), by co-finanziamento MURST 1998 (ex 40%), by CARSO Consortium Cancer Research Center, University of Bari, and AFORIGE (Associazione per la Ricerca e la Formazione in Geriatria). V.S. and A.V. participate in the Ph.D.: "Carcinogenesis, Aging, and Immunoregulation", supported by European Union.

References

1. Crook T, Bartus RT, Ferris SH et al (1986) Age-associated memory impairment: proposed diagnostic criteria and measures of clinical change – report of a National Institute of Mental Health Work Group. Dev Neuropsychol 2:261-276
2. Hanninen T, Hallikainen M, Koivisto K et al (1995) A follow-up study of age-associated memory impairment: neuropsychological predictors of dementia. J Am Geriatr Soc 43:1007-1015
3. Ritchie K, Leibovici D, Ledesert B et al (1996) A typology of subclinical senescent cognitive disorder. Br J Psychiatry 168:470-476
4. American Psychiatric Association Committee on Nomenclature and Statistics (1994) Diagnostic and statistical manual of mental disorders. 4th edn (DSM-IV). American Psychiatric Association, Washington
5. Levy R (1994) Aging-associated cognitive decline. Working Party of the International Psychogeriatrics Association in collaboration with the World Health Organization. Int Psychogeriatr 6:63-68
6. Brayne C, Calloway P (1988) Normal ageing, impaired cognitive function and senile dementia of Alzheimer type: a continuum? Lancet I:1265-1267
7. Paykel ES, Brayne C, Huppert FA et al (1994) Incidence of dementia in a population older than 75 years in the United Kingdom. Arch Gen Psychiatry 51:325-332
8. Bowen J, Teri L, Kukull W, McCormick W, McCurry SM, Larson EB (1997) Progression to dementia in patients with isolated memory loss. Lancet 349:763-765
9. Nolan KA, Blass JP (1992) Preventing cognitive decline. Clin Geriatr Med 8:19-34
10. Fillit HM (1997) The clinical significance of normal cognitive decline in late life. In: Fillit HM, Butler RN (eds) Cognitive decline. Strategies for prevention. Oxford University Press, Oxford, pp 1-7
11. Breteler MMB et al (1994) Cardiovascular disease and distribution of cognitive function in elderly people: the Rotterdam Study. BMJ 308:1604-1608
12. Launer LJ et al (1995) The association between midlife blood pressure levels and late-life cognitive function. JAMA 274:1846-1851
13. Richardson JT (1990) Cognitive function in diabetes mellitus. Neurosci Biobehav Rev 14:385-388
14. Blazer D, Burchett B, Service C, Grorge LK (1991) The association of age and depression among the elderly: an epidemiologic exploration. J Gerontol 46:M210-M215
15. Rogers RL, Meyer JS, Mortal KF (1990) After reaching retirement age, physical activity sustains cerebral perfusion and cognition. J Am Geriatr Soc 38:123-128
16. White LR, Foley DJ, Havlik RJ (1997) Lifestyle risk factors for cognitive impairment. In: Fillit HM, Butler RN (eds.) Cognitive decline. Strategies for prevention. Oxford, University Press, Oxford, pp 23-32

17. Sahyoun NR, Otradovec CL, Hartz SC et al (1988) Dietary intakes and biochemical indicators of nutritional status in an elderly, institutionalized population. Am J Clin Nutr 47:524-533
18. Goodwin J, Goodwin J, Garry P (1983) Association between nutritional status and cognitive functioning in a healthy elderly population. JAMA 249:2917-2921
19. Siebens H, Trupe E, Siebens A et al (1986) Correlates and consequences of eating dependency in institutionalized elderly. J Am Geriatr Soc 34:192-198
20. Capurso A, Solfrizzi V, Panza F et al (1997) Dietary patterns and cognitive functions in elderly subjects. Aging Clin Exp Res 9 [Suppl]:45-47
21. Solfrizzi V, Panza F, Torres F et al (1999) High monounsaturated fatty acids intake protects against age-related cognitive decline. Neurology 52:1563-1569
22. Panza F, Solfrizzi V, Colacicco AM et al (2003) Mediterranean diet and cognitive decline. Public Health Nutr (in press)
23. Amaducci L, Baldereschi M, Di Carlo A et al (1997) Prevalence of chronic diseases in older Italians: comparing self-reported and clinical diagnoses. Int J Epidemiol 26:995-1002
24. Folstein MF, Folstein SE, McHugh PR (1975) "Mini-Mental State": a practical method for grading the cognitive state of patients for the clinician. J Psychiatr Res 12:189-198
25. Spinnler H, Tognoni G (1987) Standardizzazione e taratura italiana di test neuropsicologici. Ital J Neurol Sci 6 [Suppl 8]:12-120
26. Barigazzi R, Della Sala S, Laiacona M, Spinnler H, Valenti V (1987) Esplorazione testistica della memoria di prosa. Ric Psicol 1:50-80
27. La Rue A, Koehler KM, Wayne SJ, Chiulli SJ, Haaland KY, Garry PJ (1997) Nutritional status and cognitive functioning in a normally aging sample: a 6-y reassessment. Am J Clin Nutr 65:20-29
28. Pradignac A, Schlienger M, Velten M, Mejean L (1995) Relationships between macronutrient intake, handicaps, and cognitive impairments in free living elderly people. Aging Clin Exp Res 7:67-74
29. Ortega RM, Requejo AM, Andres P et al (1997) Dietary intake and cognitive function in a group of elderly people. Am J Clin Nutr 66:803-809
30. Manna C, Galletti P, Cucciolla V, Moltedo O, Leone A, Zappia V (1997) The protective effect of the olive oil polyphenol (3,3-dihydroxyphenyl)-ethanol counteract reactive oxygen metabolite-indeced cytotoxicity in Caco-2 cells. J Nutr 127:286-292
31. Mittenberg W, Seidenberg M, O'Leary DS, Di Giulio DV (1989) Changes in cerebral functioning associated with normal aging. J Clin Exp Neuropsychol 11:918-932
32. Jama JW, Launer LJ, Witteman JC et al (1996) Dietary antioxidants and cognitive function in a population-based sample of older persons. The Rotterdam study. Am J Epidemiol 144:275-280
33. Lopez GH, Ilincheta de Boschero MG, Castagnet PI, Giusto NM (1995) Age-associated changes in the content and fatty acids composition of brain glycerophospholipids. Comp Biochem Physiol B Biochem Mol Biol 112:331-343
34. Marzo I, Martinez-Lorenzo MJ, Anel A et al (1995) Biosynthesis of unsaturated fatty acids in the main cell lineages of human leukemia and lymphoma. Biochim Biophys Acta 1257:140-148
35. Kalmijn S, Feskens EJ, Launer LJ, Kromhout D (1997) Polyunsaturated fatty acids, antioxidants, and cognitive functions in very old men. Am J Epidemiol 145:33-41
36. Swank RL (1950) Multiple sclerosis: a correlation of its incidence with dietary fat. Am J Med Sci 220:441-450
37. Swank RL, Dugan BB (1990) Effect of low saturated fat diet in early and late cases of multiple sclerosis. Lancet 336:37-39
38. Alter M, Yamoor M, Harshe M (1974) Multiple sclerosis and nutrition. Arch Neurol 31:267-272

39. Agranoff BW, Goldberg D (1974) Diet and the geographical distribution of multiple sclerosis. Lancet II:1061-1066
40. Bates D (1989) Lipids and multiple sclerosis. Biochem Soc Trans 17:289-291
41. Angulo-Guerrero O, Oliart RR (1998) Effects of dietary polyunsaturated fatty acids on rat brain plasma membrane fatty acid composition. Arch Latinoam Nutr 48:287-292
42. Fernstrom JD (1999) Effects of dietary polyunsaturated fatty acids on neural function. Lipids 34:161-169
43. Swank RL (1991) Multiple sclerosis: fat oil relationship. Nutrition 7:368-376
44. Millar JH, Zilkha KJ, Langman MJ et al (1973) Double blind trial of linoleate supplementation of the diet in multiple sclerosis. BMJ 31:765-768
45. Bates D, Fawcett PR, Shaw DA, Weightman D (1978) Polyunsaturated fatty acids in treatment of acute remitting multiple sclerosis. BMJ 2:1390-1392
46. Paty DW, Cousin HK, Read S, Adlakha K (1978) Linoleic acid in multiple sclerosis; failure to show the therapeutic benefit. Acta Neurol Scand 58:53-58
47. Bates D, Cartlidge NE, French JM et al (1989) A double blind controlled trial of long chain n-3 polyunsaturated fatty acids in the treatment of multiple sclerosis. J Neurol Neurosurg Psychiatry 52:18-22
48. Kurtzke JF (1975) Reassessment of the distribution of multiple sclerosis. Acta Neurol Scand 51:110-136
49. Esparza ML, Sasaki S, Kesteloot H (1995) Nutrition, latitude, and multiple sclerosis mortality: an ecologic study. Am J Epidemiol 142:733-737
50. Mach F, Schonbeck U, Libby P (1998) CD40 signaling in vascular cells: a key role in atherosclerosis? Atherosclerosis [Suppl] 137:S89-S95
51. Gerritse K, Laman JD, Noelle RJ et al (1996) CD40-CD40 ligand interactions in experimental allergic encephalommyelitis and multiple sclerosis. Proc Natl Acad Sci USA 93:2499-2504
52. Schoenherr WD, Jewel DE (1997) Nutritional modification of inflammatory disease. Semin Vet Med Surg (Small Anim) 12:212-222
53. Grimble RF, Tappia PS (1998) Modulation of pro-inflammatory cytokines biology by unsaturated fatty acids. Z Ernahrungswiss 37 [suppl 1]:57-65
54. Yaqoob P, Pala HS, Cortina-Borja M et al (1998) Effect of olive oil on immune function in middle-aged men. Am J Clin Nutr 67:129-135
55. Carluccio MA, Massaro M, Bonfrate C et al (1999) Oleic acid inhibits endothelial activation: a direct vascular antiatherogenic mechanism of a nutritional component in the Mediterranean diet. Arterioscler Thromb Vasc Biol 19:220-228
56. Massaro M, Carluccio MA, De Caterina R (1999) Direct vascular antiatherogenic effects of oleic acid: a clue to the cardioprotective effects of the Mediterranean diet. Cardiologia 44:507-513
57. De Andres C, Lledo A (1997) Fatty diet and multiple sclerosis. Rev Neurol 25:2032-2035
58. Chapman J, Sylantiev C, Nisipeanu P, Korczyn AD (1999) Preliminary observations on APOE e4 allele and progression of disability in multiple sclerosis. Arch Neurol 56:1484-1487
59. Chiba H (1996) Physiology and pathology of the lipid transport in the brain. Rinsho Byori 44:231-236
60. Beisiegel U, Weber W, Ihrke G, Herz J, Stanley KK (1989) The LDL-receptor-related protein, LRP, is an apolipoprotein E-binding protein. Nature 34:162-164
61. Wang X, Ciraolo G, Morris R, Gruenstein E (1997) Identification of a neuronal endocytic pathway activated by an apolipoprotein E (apoE) receptor binding peptide. Brain Res 778:6-15
62. Kowal RC, Herz J, Goldstein JL, Esser V, Brown MS (1989) Low density lipoprotein receptor related protein mediates uptake of cholesteryl esters derived from apoprotein E-enriched lipoproteins. Proc Natl Acad Sci USA 86:5810-5814

63. Gliemann J (1998) Receptors of the low density lipoprotein (LDL) receptor family in man. Multiple functions of the large family members via interaction with complex ligand. Biol Chem 379:951-964
64. Corbo RM, Scacchi R, Mureddu L, Mulas G, Alfano G (1995) Apolipoprotein E polymorphism in Italy investigated in native plasma by a simple polyacrylamide gel isoelectric focusing technique. Comparison with frequency data of other European populations. Ann Hum Genet 59:197-209
65. Gerdes LU, Klausen IC, Sihm I, Faergeman O (1992) Apoliprotein E polymorphism in a Danish population compared to findings in 45 other populations around the world. Genet Epidemiol 9:155-167
66. Panza F, Solfrizzi V, Torres F et al (1999) Decreased frequency of apolipoprotein E epsilon4 allele from Northern to Southern Europe in Alzheimer's disease patients and centenarians. Neurosci Lett 277:53-56

Neuroprotection in Acute Ischemic Stroke: Lessons for Early Treatment in Multiple Sclerosis

J. De Keyser, G. Ramsaransing, E. Zeinstra, N. Wilczak

Rationale for Neuroprotective Therapy in Acute Ischemic Stroke

A target for treatment of acute ischemic stroke is the penumbra, a territory of critically reduced blood flow between the core zone of an evolving infarction and the still sufficiently perfused brain. Unless there is early reperfusion of the ischemic area, neurons in the penumbra are destined to die in the ensuing hours to days, due to a cascade of biochemical events, the so-called ischemic cascade [1, 2]. Key steps in this cascade are uncontrolled depolarizations of neurons, build-up of extracellular glutamate, intracellular calcium overload, formation of nitric oxide and free radicals, and inflammation. Some forms of cell death in the ischemic penumbra also involve apoptosis [1, 2]. Studies in patients using positron emission tomography, combined perfusion and diffusion magnetic resonance imaging (MRI), and MR spectroscopy indicate that the penumbra in humans may remain viable for several (up to 48) hours after stroke onset [3-6].

Rationale for Neuroprotective Therapy in Multiple Sclerosis

One of the principal targets in multiple sclerosis (MS) is the oligodendrocyte. Axonal loss is also an important feature, and is considered to be the major pathological process responsible for irreversible neurological disability in patients with MS. It is thought to arise from injury secondary to inflammatory responses and demyelination [7, 8]. However, other yet unknown mechanisms may contribute, because the axonal damage is also present in normal-appearing white matter (part of which may represent downstream damage of axons traversing through remote demyelinated lesions) and appears to start in the early stages of the disease [9]. It is clear that protective therapies should focus on both neurons and oligodendrocytes. Studies in MS patients and animal models of MS suggest that toxic effects on these cells may be caused by proinflammatory cytokines (such as tumor necrosis factor-α) and interferon γ [10], an excessive release of excitatory amino acids (particularly glutamate) [11,12], and the formation of nitric oxide and free radicals [13-15]. Similar to ischemic stroke, the expression of apoptosis-associated proteins also contributes to cell death in MS [16]. Thus, there are many similarities in the biochemical events that lead to cell damage in both acute ischemic stroke and MS.

Why Were the Trials with Neuroprotective Drugs Negative in Ischemic Stroke?

Table 1 shows neuroprotective compounds that have been studied in clinical trials in patients with acute ischemic stroke. Although all these compounds showed neuroprotective properties in animal models of stroke, and results of small phase II trials were encouraging, confirmatory trials in larger study populations failed to show a clear benefit. Several aspects should be considered to explain these failures.

Table 1. List of neuroprotective drugs studied in clinical trials in acute ischemic stroke

Neuroprotective compound	Mechanism of action	Status
Nimodipine	Calcium antagonist	Abandoned (lack of efficacy)
Flunarizine	Calcium antagonist	Abandoned (lack of efficacy)
Selfotel	NMDA antagonist	Abandoned (unfavorable risk-benefit ratio)
Aptiganel (cerestat)	NMDA antagonist	Abandoned (unfavorable risk-benefit ratio)
Eliprodil	Polyamine-site blocker	Abandoned (lack of efficacy)
Clomethiazole	GABA-A receptor enhancing drug	Abandoned (lack of efficacy)
Lubeluzole	NO antagonist, sodium channel blocker	Abandoned (lack of efficacy)
Tirilazad	Free radical scavenger	Abandoned (lack of efficacy)
Ebselen	Free radical scavenger	Unknown
Fosphenytoin	Sodium channel antagonist	Abandoned (lack of efficacy)
Ganglioside GM1	Membrane constituent	Abandoned (lack of efficacy and presumed risk of Guillain Barré syndrome)
Citicoline	Membrane constituent	Abandoned (lack of efficacy)
Piracetam	Elevates cAMP levels and acts at the cell membrane	Abandoned (lack of efficacy)
Enlimomab	Murine antibody to endothelial adhesion molecule I	Abandoned (unfavorable risk-benefit ratio)
GV150526	Glycine site antagonist	Abandoned (lack of efficacy)
Magnesium sulfate	Blocks glutamate activity at the NMDA receptor	Ongoing
BMS-204352	Potassium channel opener	Halted (lack of efficacy)
Bay x 3702	5HT1A agonist	Ongoing
ZK-200775	AMPA antagonist	Abandoned (unfavorable risk-benefit ratio)
Nalmefene	Kappa opioid antagonist	Stopped (reason uncertain)
Hu23F2G	Monoclonal antibody against neutrophil CD11/CD18 cell adhesion molecule	Stopped (lack of efficacy)
Trafermin	Basic fibroblast growth factor	Stopped

First, there is the heterogeneity of the study population. Large cortical infarctions and lacunar infarction are usually grouped together, although they have a completely different prognosis [17]. Some patients have a clinically significant penumbra, whereas others have such a poor collateral circulation that there is little or no penumbra to be salvaged [18]. Thus, it is hardly surprising that no benefit is demonstrable when an operation designed to correct a particular pathophysiological disturbance is performed in a group of patients in which many do not have that disturbance.

Second, although the penumbra in humans may exist for a substantially longer period than in rodents, post hoc analyses of a number of trials suggested possible benefit in subgroups of patients treated within a shorter therapeutic time window than defined in the protocol. Typical examples are nimodipine [19], piracetam [20], and ebselen [21]. It is obvious from animal studies that the sooner the neuroprotective drug is given the better the outcome. A therapeutic effect may have been missed in studies allowing a long inclusion time.

Third, dosages of neuroprotective drugs that reduce infarct size in animals are usually associated with adverse effects, which may limit tolerable doses and prohibit their clinical use. Some side effects may even override the putative beneficial effect of a neuroprotective drug. Examples are the detrimental hemodynamic consequences of intravenous nimodipine [22] and an inflammatory reaction, causing fever, associated with the administration of enlimomab (a murine monoclonal antibody against ICAM-1) [23]. In some instances suboptimal doses were used because too much weight was given to safety aspects. This may account for the failure of lubeluzole and tirilazad, and contribute to the failure of NMDA antagonists. Normally, the action of a neuroprotective compound is dose related. Therefore it is hard to believe that a dose of 500 mg citicoline would be neuroprotective when a dose of 1,000 mg showed no effect [24]. Another problem is that fear of side effects may shorten the duration of treatment to levels that are insufficient for protecting the penumbra. For example, because of its sedative effects, clomethiazole was administered for only 24 h [25], and because of their psychomimetic effects NMDA antagonists were given as a single bolus, whereas it has been demonstrated that excitatory amino acids in the ischemic area may remain grossly elevated for at least 6 days after stroke onset [26].

Fourth, it is naive to think that stroke can be treated effectively just by the administration of a single drug. Optimal stroke unit care, where patients are treated by a multidisciplinary stroke team to prevent both the early and late complications of stroke [27], has been neglected in most neuroprotective trials. Many centers that participated in the trials did not have a stroke unit, which represent a good standard care. Another aspect is that in animal studies other factors, which may affect the extent of ischemic brain damage, such as blood pressure, body temperature, glucose concentration, and oxygenation, are all carefully controlled during the laboratory experiments. Although we know that drops in blood pressure, cardiac arrhythmias, hyperglycemia, hypoxia, and increased body temperature may aggravate cerebral damage [28], and may override any beneficial effect of neuroprotective agents [29], the management of these variables has been neglected in all stroke trials with neuroprotective agents conducted to date.

Lessons to be Learnt

The main lesson that has been learnt from clinical trials with neuroprotective drugs in acute ischemic stroke is that adequate pilot studies are essential before embarking on expensive and large-scale pivotal trials. Phase III trials should only be started after the time window, dosage, and duration of therapy that are likely to give a positive result, together with an acceptable safety profile, have been clearly established. In order to obtain information in small sample sizes of patients it is now possible to invoke combined diffusion-weighted and perfusion MRI as a surrogate parameter, to measure an effect on the penumbra [30].

Neuroprotective drugs should be administered as long as the ischemic cascade in the penumbra occurs, and this may be as long as 6 days. The dosage or duration of treatment should not be reduced below the therapeutic threshold in order to avoid side effects. Either the side effects should be acceptable, or adequate measures taken to control them, or further clinical development should be abandoned. More homogeneous sampling of patients may be accomplished by limiting selection of those with lesions of a certain location and size, and those with a perfusion/diffusion MR mismatch, indicating the existence of a salvageable penumbra.

Neuroprotective agents mainly target a specific pathway of the ischemic cascade. Because animal studies suggest that therapies using a combination of neuroprotective compounds interfering with different neurotoxic pathways have synergistic effects, treatment consisting of a carefully selected combination of neuroprotective drugs should be explored [2]. In other life-threatening conditions, such a cancer and AIDS, combination therapies are well accepted.

Implications for MS

In MS there is considerable theoretical and experimental support for the use of classical neuroprotective compounds similar to those used in stroke. These drugs may reduce the loss of oligodendrocytes, as well as diminish axonal damage. In order to achieve the best results, treatment should be implemented early in the course of the disease. The same general methodological principles mentioned for stroke also apply for clinical trials in patients with MS. In addition, there will be an important issue of long-term safety and efficacy of these drugs. In this respect, one can already predict that classical NMDA- and AMPA-type glutamate antagonists, although promising in animal models, will not find a place in the treatment of patients with MS [11, 12].

There are still many unanswered questions about the pathogenesis of MS. For example, it is still unclear whether axonal loss is exclusively related to demyelination, or whether there is a separate unrelated neurodegenerative process. A better understanding of the pathophysiological mechanisms is crucial to guide early neuroprotective management of MS, which may in the future consist of MS subtype-specific combinations of anti-inflammatory and neuroprotective drugs. Fortunately, we can use appropriate surrogate markers, such as the measurement of brain parenchymal fraction or total brain *N*-acetyl aspartate [31, 32], which may allow testing of several combinations in relatively small numbers of selected patients.

References

1. Dirnagl U, Iadecola C, Moskowitz MA (1999) Pathobiology of ischaemic stroke: an integrated view. Trends Neurosci 22:391-397
2. De Keyser J, Sulter G, Luiten PG (1999) Clinical trials with neuroprotective drugs in acute ischaemic stroke: are we doing the right thing? Trends Neurosci 22:535-540
3. Heis WD et al (1992) Progressive derangement of periinfarct viable tissue in ischemic stroke. J Cerebr Blood Flow Metab 12:193-203
4. Marchal G et al (1996) Prolonged persistence of substantial volumes of potentially viable brain tissue after stroke: a correlative PET-CT study with voxel-based data analysis. Stroke 27:599-606
5. Schwamm LH, Koroshetz WJ, Gregory Sorensen A et al (1998) Time course of lesion development in patients with acute stroke: serial diffusion- and hemodynamic-weighted magnetic resonance imaging. Stroke 29:2268-2276
6. Saunders DE, Howe FA, van den Boogaert A, McLean MA, Griffiths JR, Brown MM (1995) Continuing ischemic damage after acute middle cerebral artery infarction in humans demonstrated by short-echo proton spectroscopy. Stroke 26:1007-1023
7. Trapp BD, Peterson J, Ransohoff RM, Rudick R, Mork S, Bo L (1998) Axonal transection in the lesions of multiple sclerosis. N Engl J Med 338:278-285
8. Trapp BD, Ransohoff R, Rudick R (1999) Axonal pathology in multiple sclerosis: relationship to neurologic disability. Curr Opin Neurol 12:295-302
9. Arnold DL (1999) Magnetic resonance spectroscopy: imaging axonal damage in MS. J Neuroimmunol 98:2-6
10. Andrews T, Zhang P, Bhat NR (1998) TNF alpha potentiates IFN gamma-induced cell death in oligodendrocyte progenitors. J Neurosci Res 54:574-583
11. Pitt D, Raine CS, Werner P (2000) Glutamate excitotoxicity in a model of multiple sclerosis. Nat Med 6:67-70
12. Groom A, Zhu B, Smith T, Turski L (2000) Autoimmune encephalomyelitis ameliorated by AMPA antagonists. Nat Med 6:62-66
13. Smith KJ, Kapoor R, Felts PA (1999) Demyelination: the role of reactive oxygen and nitrogen species. Brain Pathol 9:69-92
14. Giovannoni G, Heales SJ, Land JM, Thompson AJ (1998) The potential role of nitric oxide in multiple sclerosis. Mult Scler 4:212-216
15. LeVine SM, Wetzel DL (1998) Chemical analysis of multiple sclerosis lesions by FT-IR microspectroscopy. Free Radic Biol Med 25:33-41
16. Kuhlmann T, Lucchinetti C, Zettl UK, Bitsch A, Lassmann H, Bruck W (1999) Bcl-2 expressing oligodendrocytes in multiple sclerosis lesions. Glia 28:34-39
17. Bamford J, Sandercock P, Dennis M, Burn J, Warlow C (1991) Classification and natural history of clinically identifiable subtypes of cerebral infarction. Lancet 337:1521-1526
18. Marchal G et al (1993) PET imaging of cerebral perfusion and oxygen consumption in acute ischaemic stroke: relation to outcome. Lancet 341:925-927

19. Mohr JP et al (1994) Meta-analysis of oral nimodipine trials in acute ischaemic stroke. Cerebrovasc Dis 4:197-203
20. De Deyn P, De Reuck J, Deberdt W, Vlietinck R, Orgogozo JM (1997) Treatment of acute ischemic stroke with piracetam. Members of the Piracetam in Acute Stroke Study (PASS) Group. Stroke 28:2347-2352
21. Yamaguchi T et al (1998) Ebselen in acute ischemic stroke : a placebo-controlled, double-blind clinical Trial. Stroke 29:12-17
22. Wahlgren NG, MacMahon DG, De Keyser J, Indredavik B, Ryman T (1994) Intravenous Nimodipine West European Stroke Trial (INWEST) of nimodipine in the treatment of acute stroke. Cerebrovasc Dis 4:204-210
23. Enlimomab Acute Stroke Trial Investigators (1997) The Enlimomab Acute Stroke Trial: final results. Cerebrovasc Dis 7 [Suppl 4]:18
24. Clark WM, Warach SJ, Pettigrew LC, Gammans RE, Sabounjian LA (1997) A randomized dose-response trial of citicoline in acute ischemic stroke patients. Citicoline Stroke Study Group. Neurology 49:671-678
25. Wahlgren NG et al (1999) Chlomethiazole Acute Stroke Study (CLASS): results of a randomised, controlled trial of chlomethiazole versus placebo in 1360 acute stroke patients. Stroke 30:21-28
26. Bullock R, Zauner A, Woodward J, Young HF (1995) Massive persistent release of excitatory amino acids following human occlusive stroke. Stroke 20:2187-2189
27. Stroke Unit Trialists' Collaboration (1997) Collaborative systematic review of the randomised trials of organised inpatient (Stroke unit) care after stroke. BMJ 314:1151-1159
28. Sulter G, De Keyser J (1999) From stroke unit care to stroke care unit. J Neurol Sci 162:1-5
29. Memezawa H, Zhao Q, Smith ML, Siesjo BK (1995) Hyperthermia nullifies the ameliorating effect of dizocilpine maleate (MK-801) in focal cerebral ischemia. Brain Res 670:48-52
30. Schlaug G et al (1999) The ischemic penumbra: operationally defined by diffusion and perfusion MRI. Neurology 53:1528-1537
31. Rudick RA, Fisher E, Lee JC, Simon J, Jacobs L (1999) Use of the brain parenchymal fraction to measure whole brain atrophy in relapsing-remitting MS. Neurology 53:1698-1704
32. Gonen O et al (2000) Total brain N-acetylaspartate. A new measure of disease load in MS. Neurology 54:15-19

Chapter 11

Soluble VCAM-1 Release Indicates Inflammatory Blood-Brain Barrier Pathology and Further Modulates Adhesion

B.A. Kallmann, V. Hummel, K.V. Toyka, P. Rieckmann

Cellular adhesion molecules, like VCAM-1 and ICAM-1, and their counter-receptors are involved in the adhesion of lymphocytes to endothelial cells in areas of inflammation. They are also a prerequisite for the transmigration process of immune cells into the inflamed tissue, e.g., across the blood-brain barrier (BBB) during inflammatory central nervous system (CNS) diseases [1]. Adhesion molecules can be induced by proinflammatory cytokines, like tumor necrosis factor-α (TNF-α), on various cell types, e.g., endothelial cells, macrophages, and lymphocytes [2].

In multiple sclerosis (MS), elevated levels of soluble VCAM-1 (sVCAM-1) in the serum, as well as an increased cerebrospinal fluid/serum ratio, positively correlated with disease activity and with the number and size of gadolinium-enhancing lesions on magnetic resonance imaging. These are therefore proposed as indicators of a pathologically altered BBB [3]. On the other hand, MS patients who benefit from treatment with interferon-β (IFN-β) exhibit increased sVCAM-1 levels [4].

To further investigate these apparent contradictions, we examined cultures of human cerebral endothelial cells (HCEC) and peripheral blood mononuclear cells (PBMC) under inflammatory conditions and compared their ability for cellular VCAM-1 expression and sVCAM-1 release. After stimulation with TNFα (1-10 ng/ml), VCAM-1 was expressed in a time- and dose-dependent manner on HCEC. After 72 h of culture, the number of VCAM-1-positive cells was increased from 39.8% without stimulation to 96.8% after addition of 10 ng/ml TNFα. TNFα-induced cellular VCAM-1 expression on HCEC peaked at 72 h of incubation, while sVCAM-1 release increased significantly after 144 h of incubation, when cellular expression had already declined. Consecutive release of sVCAM-1 might indicate shedding of sVCAM-1 from the cellular surface. No induction of VCAM-1 or release of sVCAM-1 was found under the same conditions in PBMC. Cerebral endothelial cells are therefore a likely source for sVCAM-1 in inflammatory diseases of the CNS [5].

Co-treatment of HCEC with TNFα and IFNβ was performed to investigate the effect of IFNβ on VCAM-1 expression and release during inflammatory processes. IFNβ (8-80 U/ml) did not induce cellular VCAM-1 on HCEC or release of its soluble form. Interestingly, co-treatment of HCEC with IFNβ further significantly increased TNFα-induced release of sVCAM-1 in a time- and dose-dependent manner, while cellular VCAM-1 expression remained unchanged.

Furthermore, we established an assay to investigate the role of cellular and sVCAM-1 for adhesion in HCEC. Adhesion of PBMC to HCEC could be significantly blocked by treating HCEC with monoclonal antibodies to VCAM-1 to a greater extent than after incubation with antibodies to ICAM-1. Pre-treatment of PBMC with recombinant sVCAM-1 at a concentration from 5 to 100 ng/ml, which is in the range of sVCAM-1 serum levels found in MS patients under IFNβ treatment, completely blocked adhesion of PBMC to HCEC under normal and inflammatory conditions [5].

Directly affecting the inflamed areas at the BBB by increasing sVCAM-1 release from cerebral endothelial cells in MS patients might be a mechanism by which IFNβ treatment exerts its immunomodulatory effects via reducing adhesion and further transmigration of lymphocytes. Furthermore, a dual role is proposed for TNFα (Fig. 1), first inducing VCAM-1 expression and cellular infiltra-

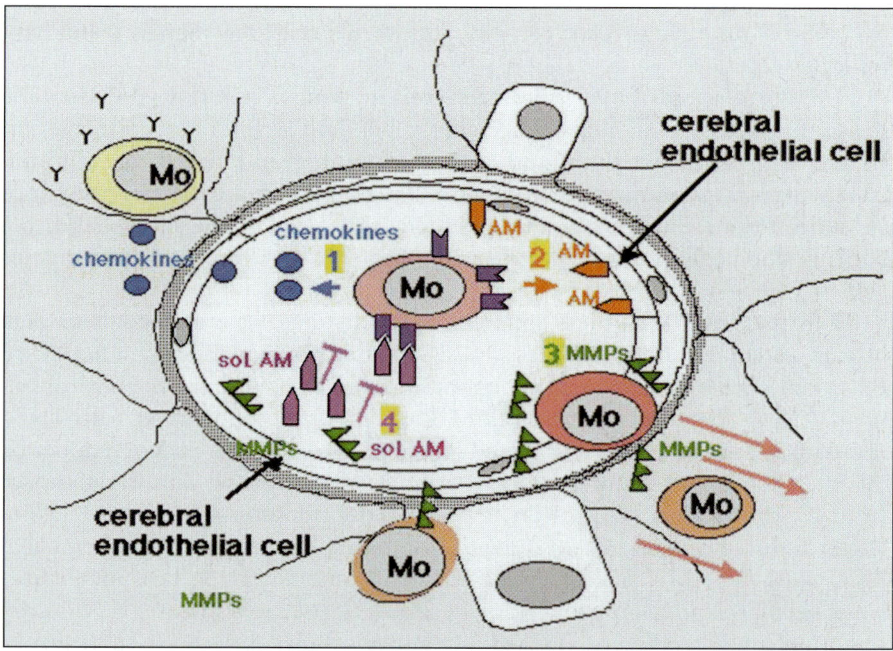

Fig. 1. Induced by inflammatory stimuli (e.g. TNFα), release of several chemokines (1) and expression of adhesion molecules (AM, e.g., VCAM-1) (2) on cerebral endothelial cells (HCEC) enhances the accumulation of a larger inflammatory infiltrate of mononuclear cells (Mo). Furthermore, matrixmetalloproteases (MMPs) (3) will be released by mononuclear cells (Mo) and HCEC causing opening and breakdown of the blood brain barrier (BBB). This is supposed to be the first proinflammatory part of the immune cascade leading to accumulation of activated immune cells beyond the BBB inducing local demyelination and axonal damage. Secreted MMPs will then enhance shedding and release of the membrane-bound adhesion molecules (e.g., soluble VCAM-1, sol. AM), introducing the second, down-regulatory (anti-inflammatory) phase by diminishing and further blocking adhesion of inflammatory cells (4)

tion into the CNS, secondary, enhancing release of sVCAM-1, thereby blocking further adhesion and downregulating immune activity.

Furthermore, HCEC were found to constitutively express matrix metalloproteases (MMP-2, MMP-3). Treatment by TNFα further upregulated MMP expression and release of MMP-3 into culture supernatants. By using the MMP inhibitor Marimastat, TNFα-induced release of sVCAM-1 was partially blocked, indicating active involvement of matrix metalloproteinases in the shedding of soluble adhesion molecules at the BBB [6] (Fig. 1).

Taken together, elevated levels of sVCAM-1 in the sera of MS patients may reflect two sides of the inflammatory process: on one hand as an indicator of disease activity during relapses, on the other as part of the initiated feedback downregulation of the inflammatory response induced by TNFα itself, and further enhanced by treatment with IFNβ. The involvement of MMPs in the shedding of soluble adhesion molecules should be considered carefully in the context of new treatment approaches in MS using MMP inhibitors.

References

1. McMurray RW (1996) Adhesion molecules in autoimmune disease. Semin Arthritis Rheum 25:215-233
2. Osborn L, Hession C, Tizard R, Vassallo C, Luhowskyj S, Chi-Rosso G, Lobb R (1989) Direct expression cloning of vascular cell adhesion molecule 1, a cytokine-induced endothelial protein that binds to lymphocytes. Cell 59:1203-1211
3. Rieckmann P, Altenhofen B, Riegel A, Baudewig J, Felgenhauer K (1997) Soluble adhesion molecules (sVCAM-1 and sICAM-1) in cerebrospinal fluid and serum correlate with MRI activity in multiple sclerosis. Ann Neurol 41:326-333
4. Rieckmann P, Altenhofen B, Riegel A, Kallmann BA, Felgenhauer K (1998) Correlation of soluble adhesion molecules in blood and cerebrospinal fluid with magnetic resonance imaging activity in patients with multiple sclerosis. Mult Scler 4:178-182
5. Kallmann BA, Hummel V, Lindenlaub T, Ruprecht K, Toyka KV, Rieckmann P (2000) Cytokine-induced modulation of cellular adhesion to human cerebral endothelial cells is mediated by soluble vascular cell adhesion molecule-1. Brain 123:687-697
6. Hummel V, Kallmann BA, Wagner S, Füller T, Bayas A, Tonn JC, Benveniste EN, Toyka KV, Rieckmann P (2001) Production of MMPs in human cerebral endothelial cells and their role in shedding adhesion molecules. J Neuropathol Exp Neurol 60:320-327

Chapter 12

Early Treatment in Multiple Sclerosis with Intravenous Immunoglobulin: Rationale and Study Design

A. ACHIRON, Y. BARAK, M. FAIBEL, S. MIRON, I. KISHNER, M. CHEN, Y. STERN, I. SAROVA-PINHAS

"... as the physicians say it happens in hectic fever, that in the beginning of the malady it is easy to cure but difficult to detect, but in the course of time, not having been either detected or treated in the beginning, it becomes easy to detect but difficult to cure."

Niccolò Machiavelli, The Prince (1640)

Introduction

Multiple sclerosis (MS) is a chronic debilitating disease that will cause significant disability to the majority of patients overtime [1]. Previous studies of the natural course of the disease showed that disability will accumulate in more that 90% of patients and additional relapses may result in significant handicap [2]. Assessment of patients with a diagnosis of probable MS with positive brain magnetic resonance imaging (MRI) demonstrated that the risk of relapsing within 1 year is 57.6% [3]. Treating patients early means treating patients with less disability. We describe the rationale for early treatment in patients with the first episode of neurological symptomatology suggestive of clinically probable MS, and the design of a randomized, double-blind, placebo-controlled trial of early treatment with intravenous immunoglobulin (IVIg, Omrix, Israel) in these patients. The primary objective of this study was to investigate the efficacy of IVIg treatment, administered at 0.4 g/kg per day for 5 consecutive days, as a loading dose, and 0.4 g/kg per day every 6 weeks thereafter as a booster dose, for a 1-year period, on the risk of patients with clinically probable MS and positive brain MRI to convert to clinically definite MS.

Early Treatment in MS – Is It Justified?

Clinical Data – Rate of Progression to Definite MS

The availability of safe and partially effective disease-modifying therapies [4-7] necessitates a change in our perspective as neurologists monitoring patients with relapsing remitting MS. It is therefore of utmost importance to make the diagnosis of MS as soon as possible, in order to be able to initiate therapy early in the course of disease.

The diagnosis of MS became easier in the last decade with the use of new neuroimaging techniques. The diagnosis of the disease is clinically determined, based on evidence for lesions disseminated over time and space. Using paraclinical tests, such as MRI of the brain and spinal cord and evoked responses, the diagnosis can be reached with the onset of the first neurological symptomatology. Once a diagnosis is established, patients should be informed, so that they will be prepared to discuss available treatment options [8]. In continuing this dialogue and making the decision which patients should be treated, risk factors associated with poor prognosis should be considered, as well as disease burden measured by brain MRI, although many of the predictors are not available at disease onset [9].

Several recent clinical trials have shown that new drug therapies can change the disease course, reduce the relapse rate, slow the progression to disability, and thus favorably affect/alter the pathological disease activity in MS [10]. The results of the Optic Neuritis Treatment Trials suggest that administration of a therapy immediately after the first attack may delay the occurrence of subsequent signs and/or symptoms and the conversion to clinically definite MS [11]. Other clinical trials in MS also indicate that better results are obtained in patients treated in the early phase of the disease [12-14]. Recently, the effect of early treatment with interferon beta-1-a on the rate of conversion from probable to clinically definite disease was evaluated in two large studies: the CHAMPS and ETOMS. Both studies demonstrated significant beneficial effect of early treatment on disease course. The results strongly support the case for early treatment, showing significant reduction in the conversion to definite MS in treated patients [15, 16].

Prospective Predictors of Conversion to Definite MS

In a recent study [3], we assessed the predictive value of different demographic and clinical variables in identifying the risk for MS patients with clinically probable diagnosis to develop definite disease. We analyzed the rate of progression to clinically definite MS in patients with the first neurological episode suggestive of MS who had a positive brain MRI compatible with the diagnosis of demyelinating disease.

We identified variables predictive of rapid progression (within 1 year) to definite MS, and found that 57.6% of patients with clinically probable MS and positive brain MRI experienced an additional relapse within 1 year. Motor involvement at onset was the only clinical parameter associated with rapid conversion to a definite diagnosis. Survival curves demonstrated that polysymptomatic involvement and a higher EDSS score at presentation correlated with rapid progression to definite diagnosis. In a similar study [2] of 224 patients at their first diagnosis of MS, a greater number of functional systems involved at onset, as well as higher residual deficits in pyramidal, visual, sphincteric, and cerebellar systems, were predictive of a poor outcome. In the relapsing-remitting subgroup, a longer first inter-attack interval was associated with a better prognosis. The presence of oligoclonal banding in the cerebrospinal fluid and a brain MRI 'strongly suggestive' or 'suggestive' of MS in the early phases of the disease were associated with a higher probability of a worse outcome.

These clinical studies suggest that the clinical activity of the disease during the early stage is strongly predictive of the subsequent evolution. As the majority of patients with probable MS and positive brain MRI will progress to clinically definite MS rapidly, and as there are only a few variables at onset to predict this rapid conversion, we suggest that all patients be treated early. To further evaluate this recommendation, we have designed the Early Treatment IVIg Trial (ET-IVIg trial) to investigate whether early treatment is clinically justified.

Immunological Evidence – Epitope Spreading

Epitope spreading is a B7-1-dependent process that plays a major pathological role in the progression of MS, and follows a hierarchical order associated with the relative encephalitogenic dominance of the myelin epitopes [17]. As a result of myelin damage and disruption of the blood-brain barrier during acute disease, T cells specific for endogenous epitopes on the same and/or different myelin proteins are primed and expand either in the periphery or locally in the central nervous system. These secondary T cells initiate an additional round of myelin destruction, leading to a clinical relapse by production of additional pro-inflammatory cytokines, similar to the bystander demyelination operative during acute disease [18]. It has been reported in both experimental autoimmune encephalomyelitis (EAE) and MS that primary proliferative autoreactivity is associated with the onset of clinical disease. The emergence of sustained secondary autoreactivity to spreading determinants is consistently associated with disease progression in both EAE and MS. Chronic progression of EAE and MS involves a shifting of autoreactivity from primary initiating self-determinants to defined cascades of secondary determinants that sustain the self-recognition process during disease progression [19]. Thus, therapeutic intervention early in MS, immediately after the onset of the autoimmune process, may be of particular importance in patients with the first episode of a demyelinating syndrome at high risk for progressing to definite MS, as it may inhibit epitope spreading and thus disease progression.

MRI Data – T1 Black Holes

It has been shown by using MRI and magnetization transfer techniques that in addition to demyelination, hypointense lesions on T1-weighted images ('black holes') relate to axonal loss. Axonal loss can occur substantially in MS, and appears early in the course of disease [20]. Moreover, even the normal-appearing white matter shows definite abnormalities with quantifiable MRI techniques. Dynamic observations demonstrate that a decrease in the concentration of *N*-acetyl aspartate, decreased magnetization transfer values and prolonged T1 relaxation time values correlate directly with axonal changes, as well as clinical disability [21-23]. In addition, the finding that patients with relapsing-remitting MS have measurable amounts of whole-brain atrophy that worsens yearly, in most cases without clinical manifestations [24], further emphasizes the need for early treatment of MS. Early treatment may limit damage to central nervous system axons or salvage injured axons and prevent the development of irreversible damage or destruction of brain parenchyma.

Cognitive Impairment

Cognitive impairment and its progression in MS have received an important place in neurological research in the last decade. Cognitive impairment in probable MS had been sparsely described. Memory loss was reported to be prevalent and associated with axonal loss and brain atrophy early in the disease course [25].

We have recently evaluated the frequency of cognitive impairment in 67 patients with probable MS, tested within a mean of one month from onset of neurological symptomatology [26]. Cognitive impairment was demonstrated in 53.7% of patients. Verbal abilities and attention span were most frequently affected. These findings suggest that between the first and second relapse, there is in fact a critical period within with pathological processes involved in cognitive impairment are not dormant, and further support the need to intervene at the earliest opportunity.

Pathological Evidence

Remyelination

Pathological studies in MS demonstrate that early demyelination can influence not only the subsequent damage, but also the potential recovery by the process of remyelination. The extent of remyelination correlates with the presence of oligodendrocytes in the lesions. Although no reliable data are available at present on the frequency of remyelination in different forms of MS, most studies agree that remyelination is especially prominent at the early stages of the disease, whereas it is sparse after several years of disease [27].

Early Axonal Loss

Pathologically, MS is characterized by inflammation. An influx of mononuclear cells occurs through a disrupted blood-brain barrier, and the secretion of a variety of inflammatory cytokines from glial cells leads to loss of myelin, disruption of oligodendrocyte integrity, and axonal loss. Transected axons are common in MS lesions, and axonal loss plays a significant role in the irreversible neurological decline of the disease [28, 29]. The decision to treat MS early should take into account these pathological events, as they affect progressive neural atrophy.

To conclude, the combined clinical and biological observations summarized so far suggest that immune abnormalities in MS can be corrected more easily during the first stages of the disease, and thus early treatments may be more effective. As immunotherapy for MS is gaining acceptance by favorably affecting the disease course, patients at an earlier stage of their disease should be treated.

It seemed to us justified to evaluate whether a treatment with an effective and well-tolerated drug can retard the long-term disability and improve the quality of life of patients who present with clinical signs and paraclinical tests that put them at high risk of developing MS.

Early Treatment with IVIg Following the First Attack of MS – a Double-Blind, Placebo-Controlled Randomized Trial

Is IVIg Treatment the Best Choice?

In designing the study and upon making a decision which drug should be used in treating patients with an early diagnosis of probable MS, we concluded that treatment with IVIg is the best choice according to the following data/criteria:

1. *Efficacy.* IVIg treatment has been shown to be effective in relapsing remitting MS patients by reducing the relapse rate, suppressing accumulating clinical disability, and decreasing the number of gadolinium (Gd)-enhancing lesions on brain MRI [30-32].
2. *Safety.* Treatment was safe without significant side-effects. A dosage of 0.4 g/kg body weight resulted in a favorable adverse events profile [33].
3. *Pregnancy and lactation.* The fact that IVIg can be safely administered during pregnancy and lactation was of utmost importance in our decision to select this drug. As the majority of patients with MS are female, and since the disease usually appears at a young age when they are interested in having children, a treatment that does not have to be discontinued before and during pregnancy has a major advantage [34, 35].
4. *Easy administration, good patient compliance.* IVIg is easily administered and probably the reason for the high rate of patient compliance is related to the relatively long periods between the IVIg boosters (6 weeks), when patients are free from medications.

Four double-blind trials in relapsing-remitting MS have demonstrated that IVIg reduces relapse rate and number of gadolinium enhancing lesions, and in this respect seems comparable to established therapies, i.e. interferon-beta and glatiramer acetate. Due to the relatively small sample size of the said studies, a meta-analysis was recently undertaken demonstrating a significant beneficial effect on the annual relapse relapse rate (effect size – 0.5; $p = 0,00003$), as well as on the proportion of relapse-free patients and progression to disability [36].

Study Period – 1 Year

Designing the study we decided to build its statistical power on a 1-year duration. This was based on our previous estimate that 57.6% of patients will have an additional attack within 1 year. Although this was a relatively high percentage, more than 40% of patients that will be treated early will not have an additional relapse. Restricting the study period to 1 year will enable us to treat them for a relatively short time.

Study Aims

The *primary outcome measures* include (1) the number of patients that will experience a second relapse within 1 year (will early treatment with IVIg prevent a second relapse?) and (2) time to reach a diagnosis of definite MS (will early treatment with IVIg delay the time to develop a second relapse?).

The *secondary outcome measures* evaluate the effect of early treatment with IVIg on: (1) MRI disease burden, (2) neurological disability (EDSS) and (3) cognitive function.

Treatment

Patients will be randomly assigned to IVIg treatment group or placebo. IVIg (Omr-IgG-am, Omrix, Israel) will be administered at a dose of 0.4 g/kg per day for 5 consecutive days (loading dose) and additional booster doses of 0.4 g/kg per day, once every 6 weeks, for a period of 1 year. Patients randomized to the placebo group will receive IV 0.9% saline in identical time schedules.

Brain MRI will be performed at study onset and at the end of the trial using a 2T MRI machine (Elscint, Israel). Data acquisition will be carried out using T2, T1, and PD pulse sequences, with Gd injection, at 3-mm slice thickness, without gap.

Statistical Calculations

The total number of patients to be enrolled in the study was calculated as 87 subjects. This estimated sample size was derived from the primary endpoint, defined as the difference in second attack prevalence between study groups, taking into consideration that equal number of patients will be enrolled for each. The following assumptions were used: (1) estimated risk for a second attack as 50%; (2) estimated treatment effect for reducing second relapse as 30%; (3) type I and type II errors for the estimation of sample size as 5% and 20%, respectively; (4) estimated drop-out rate as 3%-10%.

The study design is depicted in Fig. 1.

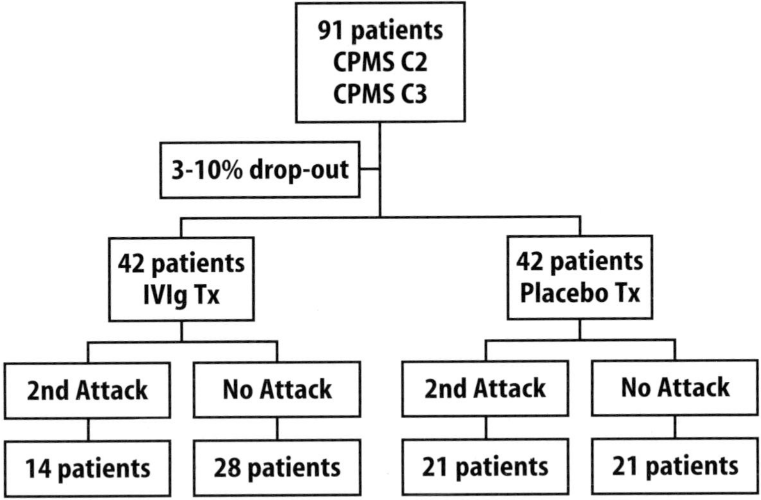

Fig. 1. Study design. *CPMS*, clinically probable multiple sclerosis

Inclusion Criteria

Inclusion criteria are: (1) age 15-50 years; (2) 3 months within the acute onset of neurological symptoms suggestive of the first attack of MS; (3) diagnosis of CPMS C2 (1 attack, 2 clinical evidences) or CPMS C3 (1 attack, 1 clinical evidence, 1 paraclinical evidence) [37]; (4) a clear regression of the neurological symptoms after the first attack, excluding a primary-progressive course; (5) positive brain MRI according to Fazekas criteria [38] with at least four focal lesions involving the white matter or three lesions if one is periventricular ($\geq$3 mm in diameter, each); (6) signed written informed consent.

Exclusion Criteria

Exclusion criteria are: (1) IgA deficiency; (2) known allergic reactions to blood products or IVIg; (3) blood tests suggestive of collagen diseases; (4) known allergic reactions to MRI contrast media.

The study is scheduled to be completed and analyzed by the end of 2003.

Conclusions

The availability of safe and effective disease-modifying therapies for MS patients, together with the immunological and pathological changes that occur early in the disease course, call for a modification in the treatment of patients presenting with the first symptomatology suggestive of MS. In deciding whom to treat, when to start treatment, and what drug to choose, it is important to consider information on disease activity acquired from clinical and MRI findings and to refer to clinical trials assessing the effect of treatment during the early phase of the disease.

References

1. Weinshenker BG (1994) Natural history of multiple sclerosis. Ann Neurol 36 [Suppl]: S6-S11
2. Amato MP, Ponziani G, Bartolozzi ML, Siracusa G (1999) A prospective study on the natural history of multiple sclerosis: clues to the conduct and interpretation of clinical trials. J Neurol Sci 168:96-106
3. Achiron A, Barak Y (2000) Multiple sclerosis – from probable to definite diagnosis: a prospective study over 7 years. Arch Neurol 57:974-979
4. Lublin FD, Whitaker JN, Eidelman BH, Miller AE, Arnason BG, Burks JS (1996) Management of patients receiving interferon beta-1b for multiple sclerosis: report of a consensus conference. Neurology 46:12-18
5. Simon JH, Jacobs LD, Campion M, Wende K, Simonian N, Cookfair DL et al (1998) Magnetic resonance studies of intramuscular interferon beta-1a for relapsing multiple sclerosis. The Multiple Sclerosis Collaborative Research Group. Ann Neurol 43:79-87
6. Wolinsky JS (1995) Copolymer 1: a most reasonable alternative therapy for early relapsing-remitting multiple sclerosis with mild disability. Neurology 45:1245-1247
7. Achiron A, Gabbay U, Gilad R, Hassin-Baer S, Barak Y, Gornish M, Elizur A, Goldhammer Y, Sarova-Pinhas I (1998) Intravenous immunoglobulin treatment in multiple sclerosis: effect on relapses. Neurology 50:398-402
8. Miller A (1998) Diagnosis of multiple sclerosis. Semin Neurol 18:309-316
9. Bourdette D, Antel J, McFarland H, Montgomery E (1999) Monitoring relapsing remitting MS patients. J Neuroimmunol 98:16-21
10. Thompson AJ, Noseworthy JH (1996) New treatments for multiple sclerosis: a clinical perspective. Curr Opin Neurol 9:187-198
11. Trials ECFWGfT (1995) Guidelines for early treatment trials in patients presenting with clinical and paraclinical abnormalities which put them at high risk for conversion to multiple sclerosis. European Charcot Foundation Working Group for Treatment Trials. Mult Scler 1 [Suppl 1]:S55-S59
12. Comi G, Barkhof F, Durelli L, Edan G, Fernandez O, Filippi M, Hartung HP, Hommes OR, Seeldrayers P, Soelberg-Sorensen P (1995) Early treatment of multiple sclerosis with Rebif (recombinant human interferon beta): design of the study. Mult Scler 1 [Suppl 1]:S24-S27
13. Munschauer FE, Stuart WH (1997) Rationale for early treatment with interferon beta-1a in relapsing-remitting multiple sclerosis. Clin Ther 19:868-882
14. Rudick RA, Goodman A, Herndon RM, Panitch HS (1999) Selecting relapsing remitting multiple sclerosis patients for treatment: the case for early treatment. J Neuroimmunol 98:22-28
15. Jacobs LD, Beck RW, Simon JH, Kinkel RP, Brownscheidle CM, Murray TJ, Simonian NA, Slasor PJ, Sandrock AW (2000) Intramuscular interferon beta-1a therapy initiated during a first demyelinating event in multiple sclerosis. CHAMPS Study Group. N Engl J Med 343:898-904
16. Comi G, Filippi M, Barkhof F, Durelli L, Edan G, Fernandez O, Hartung H, Seeldrayers P, Sorensen PS, Rovaris M, Martinelli V, Hommes OR (2001) Effect of

early interferon treatment on conversion to definite multiple sclerosis: a randomised study. Lancet 357:1576-1582

17. Vanderlugt CL, Neville KL, Nikcevich KM, Eagar TN, Bluestone JA, Miller SD (2000) Pathologic role and temporal appearance of newly emerging autoepitopes in relapsing experimental autoimmune encephalomyelitis. J Immunol 164:670-678

18. Miller SD, McRae BL, Vanderlugt CL, Nikcevich KM, Pope JG, Pope L, Karpus WJ (1995) Evolution of the T-cell repertoire during the course of experimental immune-mediated demyelinating diseases. Immunol Rev 144:225-244

19. Tuohy VK, Yu M, Yin L, Kawczak JA, Kinkel RP (1999) Spontaneous regression of primary autoreactivity during chronic progression of experimental autoimmune encephalomyelitis and multiple sclerosis. J Exp Med 189:1033-1042

20. Barkhof F, van Walderveen M (1999) Characterization of tissue damage in multiple sclerosis by nuclear magnetic resonance. Philos Trans R Soc Lond B Biol Sci 354:1675-1686

21. Matthews PM, De Stefano N, Narayanan S, Francis GS, Wolinsky JS, Antel JP, Arnold DL (1998) Putting magnetic resonance spectroscopy studies in context: axonal damage and disability in multiple sclerosis. Semin Neurol 18:327-336

22. Miller DH, Grossman RI, Reingold SC, McFarland HF (1998) The role of magnetic resonance techniques in understanding and managing multiple sclerosis. Brain 121:3-1224

23. Davie CA, Silver NC, Barker GJ, Tofts PS, Thompson AJ, McDonald WI, Miller DH (1999) Does the extent of axonal loss and demyelination from chronic lesions in multiple sclerosis correlate with the clinical subgroup? J Neurol Neurosurg Psychiatry 67:710-715

24. Rudick RA, Fisher E, Lee JC, Simon J, Jacobs L (1999) Use of the brain parenchymal fraction to measure whole brain atrophy in relapsing-remitting MS. Multiple Sclerosis Collaborative Research Group. Neurology 53:1698-1704

25. Zivadinov R, Sepcic J, Nasuelli D, De Masi R, Bragadin LM, Tommasi MA, Zambito-Marsala S, Moretti R, Bratina A, Ukmar M, Pozzi-Mucelli RS, Grop A, Cazzato G, Zorzon M (2001) A longitudinal study of brain atrophy and cognitive disturbances in the early phase of relapsing-remitting multiple sclerosis. J Neurol Neurosurg Psychiatry 70:773-780

26. Achiron A, Barak Y (2003) Cognitive impairment in probable multiple sclerosis. J Neurol Neurosurg Psychiatry 74:443-446

27. Lassmann H, Bruck W, Lucchinetti C, Rodriguez M (1997) Remyelination in multiple sclerosis. Mult Scler 3:133-136

28. Trapp BD, Peterson J, Ransohoff RM, Rudick R, Mork S, Bo L (1998) Axonal transection in the lesions of multiple sclerosis. N Engl J Med 339:278-285

29. Trapp BD, Bo L, Mork S, Chang A (1999) Pathogenesis of tissue injury in MS lesions. J Neuroimmunol 98:49-56

30. Fazekas F, Deisenhammer F, Strasser-Fuchs S, Nahler G, Mamoli B (1997) Randomised placebo-controlled trial of monthly intravenous immunoglobulin therapy in relapsing-remitting multiple sclerosis. Austrian Immunoglobulin in Multiple Sclerosis Study Group. Lancet 349:589-593

31. Sorensen PS, Wanscher B, Jensen CV, Schreiber K, Blinkenberg M, Ravnborg M, Kirsmeier H, Larsen VA, Lee ML (1998) Intravenous immunoglobulin G reduces MRI activity in relapsing multiple sclerosis. Neurology 50:1273

32. Achiron A, Gabbay U, Gilad R, Hassin-Baer S, Barak Y, Gornish M, Elizur A, Goldhammer Y, Sarova-Pinhas I (1998) Intravenous immunoglobulin treatment in multiple sclerosis: effect on relapses. Neurology 50:398-402

33. Achiron A (1997) Complications of intravenous immune globulin treatment in neurologic disease. Neurology 49:899-900

34. Achiron A, Rotstein Z, Noy S, Mashiach S, Dulitzky M, Achiron R (1996) Intravenous immunoglobulin treatment in the prevention of childbirth- associated acute exacerbations in multiple sclerosis: a pilot study. J Neurol 243:25-28
35. Orvieto R, Achiron R, Rotstein Z, Noy S, Bar-Hava I, Achiron A (1999) Pregnancy and multiple sclerosis: a 2-year experience. Eur J Obstet Gynecol Reprod Biol 82:191-194
36. Sorensen PS, Fazekas F, Lee M (2002) Intravenous immunoglobulin G for the treatment of relapsing-remitting multiple sclerosis: a meta-analysis. Eur J Neurol 9:557-563
37. Poser CM, Paty DW, Scheinberg L, McDonald WI, Davis FA, Eber GC, Johnson KP, Sibley WA, Silberberg DH, Tourtellotte WW (1983) New diagnostic criteria for multiple sclerosis: guidelines for research protocols. Ann Neurol 13:227-231
38. Fazekas F, Barkhof F, Filippi M, Grossman RI, Li DK, McDonald WI, McFarland HF, Paty DW, Simon JH, Wolinsky JS, Miller DH (1999) The contribution of magnetic resonance imaging to the diagnosis of multiple sclerosis. Neurology 53:448-456

Serial Magnetic Resonance Imaging in Patients with a First Clinical Episode Suggestive of Multiple Sclerosis: Outline of a Research Protocol

C. Pozzilli, P. Pantano, S. Di Legge, F. Caramia, M.C. Piattella, I. Pestalozza, W. Nucciarelli, A. Paolillo, L. Bozzao, G.L. Lenzi

Introduction

The application of magnetic resonance imaging (MRI) in multiple sclerosis (MS) has provided powerful insights into the evolution of the disease process over time. MRI has an established role in the diagnosis and has also been used to investigate the natural course of the disease and to monitor treatment effects in clinical trials [1].

In patients with clinically isolated syndrome (CIS) suggestive of MS, brain MRI revealed multifocal white matter abnormalities indistinguishable from MS in 50%-80% [2-5]. Previous studies have shown that such lesions at presentation can predict the risk of progression to clinically definite MS (CDMS) in the next 1-5 years [6-8]. The results of a 10-year clinical follow-up study showed that the progression to CDMS occurred in 83% of CIS patients with an abnormal brain MRI and in 11% of those with normal MRI [9]. Furthermore, the lesion load detected by T2-weighted brain MRI images at the earliest clinical stage is strongly predictive of clinical course and level of disability 10 years later [10]. The presence of gadolinium (Gd) enhancement at baseline in patients with CIS is also one of the most-predictive features of the early development of MS [5, 11].

The role of serial MRI studies in assessing the natural history of the disease and the outcome of clinical trials in relapsing-remitting (RR) MS patients was first suggested by the Bethesda group [12]. In follow-up studies performed with monthly Gd-enhanced MRI, 75% of mild RRMS patients showed more than one new enhancing lesion per month, thus indicating that the disease is active even in the clinically silent phase of the illness. Furthermore, it was also found that the frequency of the lesions was not constant and there was marked fluctuation in lesion number from month to month.

In a recent meta-analysis of longitudinal MRI studies performed on both RR and secondary progressive (SP) MS patients, the relapse rate in the 1st year was predicted by the mean number of Gd-enhancing lesions in monthly scans during the first 6 months. The best predictor for relapse rate in the subsequent 1st and 2nd year was the variation of lesion counts in the first 6-monthly scans [13].

Little is known about the natural history of disease activity in CIS patients measured by serial MRI scans. A prospective study based on serial T2-weighted and Gd-enhanced MRI at 2-month intervals for 12-15 months has been performed in seven patients with CIS [14]. Although based on a small sample, this study suggested that the presence of enhancing lesions was potentially an important prognostic measure in these patients.

Objectives

The primary aim of this research protocol is to investigate the dynamics of disease activity in a in cohort of patients with CIS and baseline MRI strongly suggestive of MS.

Longitudinal monthly Gd-enhanced MRI performed in MS patients, either in studies on natural history or in the placebo group of clinical trials, showed that MRI activity was slightly lower in SP than RRMS [13]. Whether MRI activity in the early phase of the disease is similar to, lower or higher than in CDMS is not well known.

In this serial MRI study we also investigate the evolution of brain volume changes, the outcome of new enhancing lesions to hypointense T1 lesions, and the water diffusion changes in the lesions and in the normal-appearing white matter (NAWM). These more-sophisticated MRI measures have the potential to detect more-specific pathological changes than conventional techniques but have not been explored to date in patients with CIS [1].

Furthermore, we would like to determine whether serial MRI scans may have a useful role in predicting the subsequent clinical and MRI disease activity. This information may have relevance in establishing the proper time to start a preventive treatment. Treatment has frequently been withheld from patients who do not meet the criteria of CDMS. The results of two recent multicenter trials (CHAMPS and ETOMS), however, demonstrated that a treatment with disease-modifying agents initiated at the time of the first demyelinating event delays the development of the second clinical event [15, 16]. Therefore, it should be useful to identify patients at high risk for MS who are appropriate candidates for an early treatment.

MRI criteria showing a high positive predictive value for the development of CDMS include the presence of enhancing lesions at baseline and both new T2 lesions and new enhancing lesions at an MRI follow-up performed 3 months later, indicating dissemination in space and time [5]. However, further elements should be considered in order to build a model that can better predict the conversion to CDMS. These elements may include the best timing at which MRI should be repeated after the clinical onset, and the number, location and type of new lesions at follow-up.

Trial Design and Study Population

The trial is a longitudinal 36-month study on 60 consecutive CIS patients referred to the MS Center of the University of Rome "La Sapienza". All patients are followed for the first 6 consecutive months after enrolment in the study with monthly Gd-enhanced brain MRI, standard neurological examination and disability assessment by the Expanded Disability Status Scale (EDSS) [17]. Standardized brain MRI and neurological examination are then performed at 12, 18, 24, and 36 months from the inclusion in patients who do not develop CDMS during the study. In patients who develop a second clinical relapse, the study ends at the time of the relapse, when a preventive treatment with disease-modifying agents is planned. Serial blood samples are also obtained at each study visit.

Inclusion criteria are a single clinical episode suggestive of MS and a brain MRI showing at least three typical white matter lesions according to the criteria of Fazekas et al. [18]. The first acute demyelinating event can involve the motor, sensory, visual, and the brainstem/cerebellum system. Patients with a plurisymptomatic onset suggesting a multifocal involvement of the central nervous system are also included.

Other inclusion criteria are age between 18 and 50 years (the upper limit set to reduce the likelihood of age-related non-specific abnormalities in the MRI data), no steroid-treated relapses for at least 60 days before entry in to the study (this delay may result in an underdetection of Gd-enhancing lesions at baseline scan but at the same time an interval of 2 months should minimize the effect of steroids on Gd enhancement), and written informed consent to participate in the study.

Clinical and MRI Assessment

Conversion to CDMS is defined as the occurrence of an additional relapse, disseminated in time and space, with clinical evidence on neurological examination of the new lesion. Relapses are defined according to the criteria set by Poser et al. [19]. EDSS ratings are performed by two well-trained neurologists (S.D.L., F.B.) who are not involved in any other aspect of the trial but in neurological examinations.

MRI is performed with a 1.5-T magnet (Philips Gyroscan NT 15). For all conventional brain imaging the field of view (FOV) is 24 0 cm; matrix 256 × 256, and number of excitations (NSA) 2. Proton density and T2-weighted conventional spin-echo (CSE) images (TR=2,000 ms, TE=20/90 ms), fluid-attenuated inversion-recovery (FLAIR) images (TR=6,000 ms, TE=150 ms), and T1-weighted spin echo imaging (TR=550 ms, TE=12 ms) are acquired in the axial plane with 5-mm contiguous slices. The T1-weighted enhanced images of the brain are obtained before and after injection of an intravenous bolus of 0.3 mmol/kg Gd-DTPA [20]. Diffusion-weighted (DWI) images are acquired using a multi-slice, single-shot spin-echo EPI sequence. Time acquisition is 36 s. The following parameters are used: TR=6,000, TE=34, flip angle=90, EPI factor=63, bmax=1,000, three orthogonal directions=PMS, slices=20, slice thickness=5 mm, slice gap=0 mm, image matrix=128×128, and FOV=240 mm. Apparent diffusion coefficient (ADC) maps are then calculated on the isotropic DWI images (trace).

MRI Analysis

Lesions are counted and marked on the hard copies of each scan by an experienced radiologist (M.C.P.). The following MRI measures will be taken into account for the analysis:

Number of newly "active lesions" as seen on T2-weighted and Gd-enhanced monthly brain MRI and display one of the following features:

- new Gd-DTPA enhancement on T1-weighted scan
- non-enhancing on T1-weighted scan but new on T2-weighted scan
- non-enhancing on T1-weighted scan but showing new enlargement on T2-weighted scan.

Number of "active scans" (i.e., containing at least one new "active lesion").

Number of "active patients" (i.e., patients with "active scans").

Total number of persistent "active lesions" as seen on T2-weighted and Gd-enhanced monthly brain MRI.

Number of lesions on T2-weighted scans, on enhanced and unenhanced T1-weighted scans at entry and at 6, 12, 18, 24, and 36 months.

Number of new or enlarging lesions as seen on T2-weighted scans. Number of active T2-weighted scans (i.e., containing new or enlarged lesions).

Total lesion volume (TLV) and infratentorial lesion volume (ILV) on unenhanced and enhanced T1, T2-weighted, and FLAIR weighted scans measured at each scan by a semiautomated contouring program (DispImage, D. Plummer, UCL Hospitals Trust).

The presence of lesions in five prespecified regions of the brain is recorded: (1) infratentorial lesions, (2) periventricular lesions, (3) subcortical/cortical (at the gray matter junction) lesions, (4) discrete (neither periventricular nor cortical/subcortical), and (5) lesions in the corpus callosum.

Quantification of MRI brain volume is assessed using dedicated software for a brain parenchyma segmentation, based on signal intensity tresholding. The measurement is performed at entry and at 6, 12, 18, 24, and 36 months.

ADC values are calculated in both lesions and NAWM and ADC changes are evaluated over time.

References

1. Miller DH, Grossmann RI, Reingold SC, McFarland HF (1999) The role of magnetic resonance techniques in understanding and managing multiple sclerosis. Brain 121:3-1224

2. Jacobs L, Kinkel PR, Kinkel WR (1986) Silent brain lesions in patients with isolated idiopathic optic neuritis. A clinical and nuclear magnetic resonance imaging study. Arch Neurol 43:452-455

3. Ormerod IE et al (1987) The role of NMR imaging in the assessment of multiple sclerosis and isolated neurological lesions. A quantitative study. Brain 110:1579-1616

4. Ford B, Tampieri D, Francis G (1992) Long-term follow-up of acute partial transverse myelopathy. Neurology 42:250-252

5. Brex PA et al (1999) Multisequence MRI in clinically isolated syndromes and the early development of MS. Neurology 53:1184-1190

6. Morrissey SP et al (1993) The significance of brain magnetic resonance imaging abnormalities at presentation with clinically isolated syndromes suggestive of multiple sclerosis. A 5-year follow-up study. Brain 116:135-146

7. Beck RW et al (1993) The effect of corticosteroids for acute optic neuritis on the subsequent development of multiple sclerosis. The Optic Neuritis Study Group. N Engl J Med 329:1764-1769

8. Filippi M et al (1994) Quantitative brain MRI lesion load predicts the course of clinically isolated syndromes suggestive of multiple sclerosis. Neurology 44:635-641

9. O'Riordan JI et al (1998) The prognostic value of brain MRI in clinically isolated syndromes of the CNS. A 10-year follow-up. Brain 121:495-503

10. Sailer M et al (1999) Quantitative MRI in patients with clinically isolated syndromes suggestive of demyelination. Neurology 52:599-606

11. Barkhof F et al (1997) Comparison of MRI criteria of first presentation to predict conversion to clinically definite multiple sclerosis. Brain 120:2059-2069

12. McFarland HF et al (1992) Using gadolinium-enhanced magnetic resonance imaging lesions to monitor disease activity in multiple sclerosis. Ann Neurol 32:758-766

13. Kappos L et al (1999) Predictive value of gadolinium-enhanced magnetic resonance imaging for relapse rate and changes in disability or impairment in multiple sclerosis: a meta-analysis. Gadolinium MRI Meta-analysis Group. Lancet 353:964-969

14. Kinkel RP, Simon JH, Baron B (1999) Bimonthly cranial MRI activity following an isolated demyelinating syndrome: potential outcome measures for future multiple sclerosis 'prevention' trials. Mult Sci 5:307-312

15. Jacobs LD, Beck RW, Simon JH et al (2000) Intramuscular interferon beta 1a-therapy initiated during a first demyelinating event in multiple sclerosis. N Engl J Med 343:898-904

16. Comi G, Filippi M, Barkhof F et al (2001) Effect of early interferon treatment on conversion to definite multiple sclerosis: a randomised study. Lancet 357:1576-1582

17. Kurtzke JF (1983) Rating neurologic impairment in multiple sclerosis: an expanded disability status scale (EDSS). Neurology 33:1444-1452

18. Fazekas F et al (1988) Criteria for an increased specificity of MRI interpretation in elderly subjects with suspected multiple sclerosis. Neurology 38:1822-1825

19. Poser CM et al (1983) New diagnostic criteria for multiple sclerosis: guidelines for research protocols. Ann Neurol 13:227-231

20. Filippi M et al (1998) A multi-centre longitudinal study comparing the sensitivity of monthly MRI after standard and triple dose gadolinium-DTPA for monitoring disease activity in multiple sclerosis. Implications for phase II clinical trials. Brain 21:2011-2020

T1-Hypointense Lesions (T1 Black Holes) in Mild-to-Moderate Disability Relapsing Multiple Sclerosis

J.H. Simon, L. Jacobs, N. Simonian, and the MS Collaborative Research Group

Introduction

T1-hypointense lesions (T1-black holes) in multiple sclerosis (MS) are areas of relatively severe central nervous system (CNS) damage compared with the more non-specific T2-hyperintense lesions, which show greater signal intensity than normal brain on T2-weighted magnetic resonance imaging (MRI). The T1-hypointense lesions are areas of axonal loss, as well as matrix disruption [1, 2]. T1-hypointense lesions are moderately correlated with focal reduction in the magnetization transfer index [3, 4] and reduced N-acetylaspartate (NAA) [2]. T1-hypointense lesions appear to evolve from only a subset of prior enhancing MS lesions. Recent studies have suggested that an increase in T1-hypointense lesions is more strongly correlated with progression of disability in secondary progressive MS than T2-hyperintense lesions [5, 6]. For these reasons, the T1-hypointense lesions are considered to be potential independent markers of the MS disease process compared with the conventional MR measures of subclinical disease – the T2-lesions, and markers of inflammation, the enhancing lesions [7, 8]. Here we summarize the analyses of T1-black holes from the MS Collaborative Research Group Trial of interferon β-1a, which provided an opportunity to determine the natural history of T1-black holes in relatively early MS, in patients with only mild-to-moderate disability, and to evaluate the potential of T1-black holes as a measure of treatment efficacy. Details of this work have been published previously [9].

Patients and Methods

Patients

Patients were from the Phase III Multiple Sclerosis Collaborative Research Group (MSCRG) trial of interferon β-1a (Avonex) [10]. Patients were randomized to receive either placebo or 30 µg (6 million IU) of interferon β-1a (Avonex, Biogen) once weekly by intramuscular injection. The mean age of the T1-hypointense lesion study group was 36.3 years (SD 6.9), the expanded disability status scale (EDSS) range for entry was 1.0 to 3.5, with a mean of 2.3 (SD 0.8), and the mean duration of disease was 6 years (SD 5.2).

MR Imaging

The analyses were based on a subset of the full study population [9] and included 160 baseline (80 placebo, 80 interferon β-1a-treated patients) and 160 2-year MR studies. T1-hypointense lesions were determined by predefined criteria [9], including sharply demarcated regions that did not correspond to enhancing areas on T1-weighted images, to enrich for chronic T1-hypointense lesions. The T2-lesion volume at entry was a median of 12.1 ml (mean 14.9 ml, SD 15.3 ml, range 0.1-104 ml); 54% of the patients had one or more enhancing lesions at baseline. Methods for analyses of T2-hyperintense lesions and atrophy have been reported previously [9, 11, 12].

Results

Baseline Results

There were no significant differences in the treatment groups for any of the baseline clinical or MRI characteristics. The median T1-hypointense lesion volume was 0.64 ml (mean 1.5 ml, SD 2.0 ml, range 0-12.4 ml). There was a strong correlation at baseline between T1-hypointense lesion volume and T2-hyperintense lesion volume ($r = 0.8$, $p <0.001$). Significant correlations were seen between T1-hypointense lesions and ventricle and corpus callosum atrophy measures ($|r| = 0.34\text{-}0.46$, $p < 0.0010$), and for T1- hypointense lesions and enhancing lesion volume at baseline ($r = 0.25$, $p = 0.001$). The correlation between EDSS and T1-hypointense lesions was 0.22 ($p = 0.005$), nearly identical to the correlation between EDSS and T2-hyperintense lesion volume reported previously from this trial ($r = 0.22$, $p = 0.005$) [11]. There was no correlation between the ratio of T1 to T2 lesion volume (T1/T2) and EDSS or disease duration.

On-Trial Results

A small correlation was observed between the actual and percentage 2-year change in T1-hypointense lesions and change in EDSS at 2 years ($r = 0.28\text{-}0.29$, $p = 0.012$). A modest correlation was noted for T1-hypointense lesions and the cumulative number of relapses ($r = 0.34$, $p = 0.002$). Moderate correlations ($r \geq 0.36$, $p \leq 0.002$) were seen on trial between change in T1-lesion volume and enhancing lesions, new and enlarging T2-hyperintense lesions, and for change in T2-hyperintense lesion volume and change in third ventricle width ($r = 0.36$, $p = 0.002$).

In the placebo arm, for patients with enhancing lesions at baseline (GD+) , there was a 34% 2-year increment in T1-hypointense lesion volume ($p = 0.002$), which was fourfold greater than for placebo patients without enhancing lesions at baseline (GD–), whose increase as a subgroup was not significant.

Treatment Group Analyses

For the placebo patients, the median increment in T1-hypointense lesions was 0.125 ml over 2 years. This 29.1% increase from baseline was significant ($p < 0.001$). The 11.8 % median increase over 2 years for the interferon β-1a-treated patients was only 0.04 ml, which was not a significant change. Although suggestive of a treatment effect, the treatment group differences at 2 years did not reach statistical significance ($p = 0.065$). For both the GD+ and GD– groups, the increase in T1-hypointense lesions was smaller with treatment. In the interferon β-1a-treated groups, no significant baseline increment in T1-lesion volume was detected in either the GD+ or GD– groups.

Discussion

There are several results from this study. First, we find that T1-hypointense lesions are found in the majority of patients (95%) with only mild-to-moderate disability relapsing MS, and in many cases involve a large volume of white matter. There is a progressive increase in these T1-hypointense lesions over a 2-year study interval. There are indications that treatment has a favorable influence in slowing the accumulation of these relatively destructive lesions, both in the full study group, as well as in the patients with the most-active disease defined by enhancing lesions.

We have found some correlation between disability and T1-hypointense lesions, and change in disability and T1-hypointense lesion volume over 2 years. Although these correlations are only weak, the on-trial 2-year changes are stronger than for T2-hyperintense lesion change and EDSS. The relatively poor correlation overall between the MR marker and the clinical expression is no longer unexpected – the MR measures are biological markers and measures of pathophysiology, while the clinical measures (relapse and disability), are highly dependent on a complex interaction of anatomical location, lesion severity, and possibly neuronal pathway redundancy and plasticity. The correlation between T1-hypointense lesions and other measures of tissue damage, such as atrophy and the relationship to prior enhancing lesions, suggests that the T1-black holes are important biological markers of the destructive MS process, which is largely subclinical in the early stages of the disease.

Compared with the T1-hypointense lesion burden in these relapsing MS patients, patients in the earliest stages of demyelinating disease, such as those in the CHAMPS trial with a first (monosymptomatic) neurological event and a positive MRI, have a far smaller, although not insignificant, prevalence of T1-hypointense lesions. T1-hypointense lesions occur in about 50% of these patients, and the overall volume of these lesions is considerably smaller [13].

Immunomodulatory therapy with 30 μg of interferon β-1a (Avonex), administered once weekly, retards the development of T1-hypointense lesions, proportionate to or exceeding that seen in the same trial for T2-hyperintense lesion volume, new and enlarging T2-hyperintense lesions, and enhancing lesions [10, 11]. This suggests that with a more-optimal sample size T1-hypointense may be a robust and important outcome measure. Treatment with interferon β-1a appears to impede the development of both T1-hypointense and T2-hyperintense lesions. In theory these MR-based displays of pathophysiology may be uncoupled, such that treatment might decrease the non-specific T2-hyperintense lesions, yet might not retard the more-damaging effects of MS, as indicated by T1-hypointense lesions. This does not appear to be the case in this trial.

Finally, although an over-simplification, these data lend further support to the existence of two patients groups, a fast-track or aggressive group with greater risk for damage over an interval of years and a slower track, relatively less-active MS patient group [9, 11, 12]. These groups can be identified, albeit imperfectly, by a single enhanced MRI study. The patients with enhancing lesions would be expected to be at greatest risk for future disease, which may remain largely subclinical over short intervals. However, more-aggressive monitoring and treatment may be indicated to preclude further impairment, or possibly entry into the progressive stages of MS. Treatment group comparisons for the enhancing and non-enhancing populations suggest that treatment brings the most-active disease patients to the range of MR outcomes observed in patients with less-active disease, who showed less change over the study interval. These generalizations regarding activity trends are based on population studies, and should not be extrapolated to the individual patient.

Acknowledgements. Supported in part by National Institutes of Health grant NINDS R01-26321 and Biogen, Cambridge, Mass., USA.

References

1. van Walderveen MA, Kamphorst W, Scheltens P et al (1998) Histopathologic correlate of hypointense lesions on T1-weighted spin-echo MRI in multiple sclerosis. Neurology 50:1282-1288
2. van Walderveen MA, Barkhof F, Pouwels PJW et al (1999) Neuronal damage in T1-hypointense multiple sclerosis lesions demonstrated in vivo using proton magnetic resonance spectroscopy. Ann Neurol 46:79-87
3. Loevner LA, Grossman RI, McGowan KN, Cohen JA (1995) Characterization of multiple sclerosis plaques with T1-weighted MRI and quantitative magnetization transfer. AJNR 16:1473-1479
4. van Waesberghe JH, Casteijns JA, Scheltens P, Truyen L, et al (1997) Comparison of four potential MR parameters for severe tissue destruction in multiple sclerosis lesions. Magn Reson Imaging 15:155-162
5. Truyen L, van Waesberghe JHTM, Barkoff et al (1996) Accumulation of hypointense lesions ("blackholes") on T1 spin echo MRI correlates with disease progression in multiple sclerosis. Neurology 47:1469-1476
6. van Walderveen MA, Barkhof F, Hommes OR et al (1995) Correlating MRI and clinical disease activity in multiple sclerosis: relevance of hypointense lesions on short-TR/short TE (T1 weighted) spin echo images. Neurology 45:1684-1690

7. Miller DH, Albert PS, Barkhof F et al (1996) Guidclines for the use of magnetic resonance techniques in monitoring the treatment of multiple sclerosis. Ann Neurol 39:6-16

8. Simon JH (1997) Contrast enhanced MR imaging in the evaluation of treatment response and prediction of outcome in multiple sclerosis. J Magn Reson Imaging 7:29-37

9. Simon JH, Lull J, Jacobs LD et al (2000) A longitudinal study of T1 hypointense lesions in relapsing MS. Results from the MSCRG Trial of interferon beta-1a. Neurology 2000 55:185-192

10. Jacobs LD, Cookfair DL, Rudick RA et al (1996) Intramuscular interferon beta-1a for disease progression in relapsing multiple sclerosis. Ann Neurol 39:285-294

11. Simon JH, Jacobs LD, Campion M (1998) Magnetic resonance studies of intramuscular interferon b-1a for relapsing multiple sclerosis. Ann Neurol 43:79-87

12. Simon JH, Jacobs L, Campion M et al (1999) A longitudinal study of brain atrophy in relapsing MS. Neurology 53:139-148

13. CHAMPS Study Group (2002) Baseline MRI characteristics of patients at high risk for multiple sclerosis: results from the CHAMPS trial. Multiple Sclerosis 8:330-338

Acute Monosymptomatic Optic Neuritis: Potential Clues to Early Therapy in Multiple Sclerosis

D.I. KAUFMAN

Introduction

The optic nerve is a 50 mm by 4.5 mm white matter tract of the central nervous system (CNS). Its physiology and response to therapy can be precisely quantified by a number of common, easily available, neuro-ophthalmological techniques. Detection of an early, subtle, optic neuropathy is relatively easy compared with many of the difficult-to-document sensory or even motor complaints in early multiple sclerosis (MS).

Optic neuritis (ON) is an inflammatory disorder of the optic nerve. Although ON can occasionally be associated with a variety of systemic or ocular disorders, most cases are idiopathic or associated with MS. ON is the most-common acute optic neuropathy in adults under the age of 46 years. Among high-risk populations for MS, the frequency of ON is similar, about 3 per 100,000 population per year, whereas in other areas the frequency is about 1 per 100,000 population per year [1-13].

Acute ON often presents as an isolated clinical event without contributory systemic abnormalities (monosymptomatic ON). Clinical symptoms include periocular pain, abnormal visual acuity and fields, reduced color vision, afferent pupillary defect, and abnormal visual evoked potentials. The fundus may appear entirely normal or demonstrate edema of the optic nerve head (papillitis) [12-18] (Table 1).

Table 1. Features of typical acute monosymptomatic optic neuritis

1. Visual symptoms of recent onset
2. Progressive loss of vision over several days
3. Periocular pain particularly with eye movement
4. Abnormal visual acuity
5. Abnormal color vision
6. Abnormal visual field, consistent with optic neuropathy
7. Afferent pupillary defect in the eye with the abnormal function
8. Fundoscopy demonstrates optic disc edema (due to papillitis) or a normal optic nerve without atrophy
9. Age in the later teens to mid forties
10. No evidence of a contributory systemic illness associated with optic neuropathy with the exception of multiple sclerosis
11. No history of a previous optic neuritis or other optic neuropathy

Magnetic resonance imaging (MRI) white matter abnormalities identical to those seen in MS are found in up to 50%-70% of monosymptomatic ON cases [19-23]. The visual deficit of ON may worsen over 1 or 2 weeks and usually begins improving over the next month. Lack of improvement in visual function by 30 days is unusual. However, most patients have at least some residual visual function deficit, even if visual acuity improves to 20/20 [1-18]. Differential diagnosis includes compressive, ischemic, hereditary, toxic, or other inflammatory optic neuropathies (e.g., sarcoid). However, these conditions usually do not exhibit the same clinical pattern (Table 1) or rate of recovery as monosymptomatic ON [1-13].

Use of steroids in acute monosymptomatic ON has been well researched. There are various dosages that have been investigated with various routes of adminstration. These will be outlined below. In addition, use of higher-dose intravenous methylprednisolone (1 g daily for 3 days) at the onset of acute monosymptomatic ON and other similar demyelinating events followed by interferon β 1-a (IFN β 1-a) versus placebo has also been evaluated in clinical studies, and will be discussed below.

Literature Review

Treatment of monosymptomatic ON has included oral, retrobulbar, and intravenous steroids, immunoglobulin, and acupuncture [24-78]. Although there are multiple studies investigating therapy in ON, most have limitations based on design flaws or recruitment of insufficient numbers of patients. The Optic Neuritis Treatment Trial (ONTT) study group has published several papers on various aspects of this National Eye Institute-sponsored, multi-center study [11, 12, 61-81]. The ONTT enrolled 457 patients with acute ON, aged 18-46 years, and followed them for 6 months or longer [61]. The study then followed 388 ON patients (with no prior history of MS) for 5 years [79, 81]. The data revealed that oral prednisone at 1 mg/kg per day (previously the most-common method of treating ON) was no longer an appropriate therapy because it did not increase the level of visual recovery nor did it increase the speed of recovery compared with placebo [61, 62]. In addition, prednisone increased the recurrence rate of ON [61, 63, 64, 83-87].

All ONTT patients were randomized into three treatment groups: (1) oral prednisone alone (1 mg/kg per day) for 14 days (oral treatment group), (2) intravenous methylprednisolone sodium succinate 250 mg four times per day for 3 days in a hospital, followed by oral prednisone (1 mg/kg per day) for 11 days as an outpatient [intravenous treatment group (IVMP)], or (3) oral placebo for 14 days (placebo group). A placebo intravenous group was not included because study organizers could not justify, ethically or financially, hospitalizing patients for 3 days of sham intravenous therapy [67, 81].

MRI was performed in nearly all patients at study entry. Lumbar puncture was optional and performed in 133 of 457 (29.1%) of the cohort. Visual evoked potentials (VEP) were not included. All patients were treated within 8 days of symptom onset. The study was designed to determine speed and level of recovery and complications of therapy. Visual acuity, visual fields, contrast sensitivity, and color vision were measured at study entry and at seven follow-up visits during the first 6 months, at 1 year, and then annually for 5 years [67, 81].

Of the 457 patients 2 were eventually discovered to have compression as the etiology of the ON. The intravenous treatment group started to recover vision sooner than did the other two groups. By 30 days after study entry, differences between groups in vision were minimal. At 6 months there were no significant differences in visual acuity in the three treatment groups [61]. After 12 months of follow-up, visual acuity in the eye with ON at entry was better than 20/20 in 69% and 20/200 or worse in only 3% [72]. The only predictor of a poor visual outcome was poor visual acuity at study entry. Of 160 eyes starting at 20/200 or worse, only 8 (5%) were still 20/200 or worse at 6 months [12, 61, 69].

Recurrent ON was greater in the group treated with oral prednisone alone than in the other two groups [61, 63, 64]. This finding was not without controversy [83-87]. However, by year 2, 30% of patients in the with oral treatment group experienced at least one new attack of ON in *either eye* compared with 16% in the placebo group and 13% in the intravenous treatment group [61, 73, 77]. This difference continued throughout the 5-year follow-up period (41% recurrences in the prednisone treatment group and 25% in the intravenous and placebo groups) and remained highly statistically significant ($p=0.004$) for prednisone compared with placebo [80, 82].

In the 388 patients without a history of probable or definite MS at entry, brain MRI was the most-powerful predictor of the development of clinically definite MS (CDMS) within the subsequent 5 years of follow-up (Tables 2, 3 and 4) [20, 80]. Among patients with a normal MRI ($n=202$), the probability of developing CDMS within 5 years was 16%; among patients with one or two signal abnormalities ($n=61$), 37% developed CDMS and among patients with three or more white matter lesions ($n=89$), 51% [20, 80].

Soderstrom's group, in 1998, published a study of 147 patients with ON using MRI, cerebral spinal fluid (CSF), and HLA findings to determine the prognosis for MS; 116 had MRI, 146 had HLA analysis, and 143 had a lumbar puncture. These authors noted that the presence of three or more white matter lesions on MRI and the presence of oligoclonal bands in the CSF were strongly associated with the development of MS ($p<0.001$). Of 41 ON patients with oligoclonal IgG bands in the CSF, 20 had no lesions on brain MRI. Of these 20 patients, 5 went on to develop MS, even in a relatively short follow-up period [60]. In the ONTT, the predictive value of oligoclonal bands was assessed in 76 patients at 5 years and found to be very highly associated with the development of MS ($p=0.02$). However, the ONTT results suggested that CSF analysis is only useful in the risk assessment when brain MRI is normal [21].

Independent of brain MRI and CSF analysis, in the ONTT population of patients previous non-specific neurological symptoms were also predictive of the

Table 2. Cumulative probability of patients with clinically definite multiple sclerosis after specific time intervals by treatment group [74]

		Treatment group		
	Time after entry	IV methylpred (*n*=133)	Prednisone (*n*=129)	Placebo (*n*=126)
	6 months	3%	7%	7%
	1 year	6%	10%	13%
	2 years	8%	16%	18%
	3 years	18%	25%	21%
	4 years	25%	28%	26%
	5 years	27%	32%	31%
			Relative risk (95% CI)	*p* palue
2 years				
	IV vs. placebo		0.34 (0.16-0.74)	*p* = 0.006
	Prednisone vs. placebo		0.90 (0.48-1.71)	*p* = 0.75
5 years				
	IV vs. placebo		0.81 (0.50-1.30)	*p* = 0.38
	Prednisone vs. placebo		1.05 (0.67-1.65)	*p* = 0.85

[a] excludes patients with probable or definite multiple sclerosis at time of study entry
IV, intravenous therapy with methylprednisolone, 250 mg every 6 h for 3 days followed by prednisone
Prednisone, oral prednisone therapy 1 mg/kg per day for II days followed by a 4-day taper

Table 3. Cumulative probability of clinically definite multiple sclerosis after specific time intervals according to baseline magnetic resonance imaging (MRI)[a] [74]

	Baseline MRI		
Time after entry	Normal[b] (*n*=202)	1-2 abnormal signals (*n*=60)	3 or more abnormal signals (*n*=89)
6 months	1%	7%	17%
1 year	3%	14%	25%
2 years	5%	20%	31%
3 years	9%	27%	45%
4 years	14%	31%	50%
5 years	16%	37%	51%

Rate ratios and 95% confidence intervals (CI) for development of clinically definite multiple sclerosis by 2 years are:

	Rate ratio (95% CI)	*p* palue
Normal vs. 1-2 abnormal signals	2.61 (1.48-4.60)	*p* = 0.0009
Normal vs. >2 abnormal signals	4.44 (2.79-7.09)	*p* = 0.0001

[a] excludes patients with probable or definite multiple sclerosis at time of study entry
[b] includes patients with non-specific MRI changes

Table 4. Cumulative probability of developing clinically definite multiple sclerosis within 2 years of study entry according to treatment group and baseline MRI [51][a]

Baseline brain MRI	IV methylprednisolone (n=119)	Placebo (n=113)	Prenisone (n=119)
Normal+	3	3	8
1-2 signal abnormalities	15	22	23
>3 signal abnormalities	16	39	38

+ Includes non-specific changes
[a] The numbers are too small to give rate ratios, confidence intervals, and p values

development of CDMS. Lack of pain, the presence of severe optic disc swelling and mild visual acuity loss were features of the ON associated with a low risk of CDMS at 5 years in patients with no brain MRI lesions and no history of neurological symptoms or ON in the fellow eye. Age and gender were not of prognostic value. Patients with severe disc swelling, especially if associated with hemorrhages or a macular star, had no progression to CDMS over 5 years [80-82].

The intravenous treatment part of the ONTT was single masked [73]. It is doubtful that neurologists examining patients months or years after therapy, using a detailed and standardized protocol, would be biased in reporting attacks of demyelination in the IVMP group or any of the three treatment [78]. Furthermore, all forms were reviewed in a masked, independent fashion by an authority in MS [78]. The ONTT noted IVMP was associated with a reduced risk of developing CDMS in patients with an abnormal brain MRI at study entry for 2 years compared with the two other groups [73, 80]. The therapeutic effect of IVMP was no longer significant by the 3rd year of follow-up [77, 80]. Among those with a normal MRI, the 2-year rate of MS was so low that a benefit from intravenous treatment could not be established (Tables 2-4).

Herishanu's study in 1989 suggested ON conversion to MS was greater with the use of IVMP. However, this group evaluated a total of 26 patients divided into three groups with either no therapy, prednisone, or IVMP. In addition to the very low numbers for each group under analysis, the study was retrospective and the patients were not randomized [40].

Seven other ON treatment trials using corticosteroids were identified [30-33, 39, 56-59]. All were prospective, randomized, and placebo controlled. Regrettably, the small sample size in each of these studies limited their individual power to detect a clinically important treatment trend [88]. However, taken together there are some important findings. In 1969, Rawson et al. [30, 31] suggested speed of recovery was faster in patients receiving adrenocorticotropic hormone over placebo. Both this study and Bowden's demonstrated that acuity was the same at 12 months. Retrobulbar triamcinolone increased speed of recovery, but provided no improvement over placebo at 12 months [33].

Two other placebo-controlled studies used IVMP. Kapoor et al. [56] in 1998 showed there was no effect on the final visual outcome in 66 individuals with ON lesions involving the optic canal. In 1999, Wakakura et al. [13, 58] evaluated 66 patients with 500 mg of IVMP or placebo. They concluded this therapy improved the speed of recovery, but at 1 year was no better than placebo. Two oral methylprednisolone studies were reported; the Tubingen study testing 50 patients [57] and the Sellebjerg group testing 60 patients [59]. These studies used 100 mg and 500 mg oral methylprednisolone, respectively, for several days. In both there was increased speed of visual recovery, but no long-term improvement over placebo. The Sellebjerg study reported there was no increase in recurrence of ON at 1 year using oral methylprednisolone, an important finding given the ONTT results using lower-dose oral prednisone [61]. However, Sellebjerg's article also stated: "The number of patients is too low to rule out an effect on subsequent disease activity" [59].

Other publications include reports from the early 1950s dealing with gluco-corticoid treatment of ON [24, 27]. These studies used a variety of different strategies. All had serious methodology flaws, especially related to very low patient numbers, retrospective analysis, no randomization, or total lack of placebo control [88]. In a 1988 publication, Spoor and Rockwell [41] showed a very rapid recovery of vision in his 12 patients given 1 or 2 g of IVMP, some within 24 h. Unfortunately this study was neither randomized or placebo con-trolled [41]. A study by Alejandro et al. [55] in 1994 looked at 8 patients given IVMP versus 8 given oral prednisone and found no difference between groups. Other similar small studies evaluating ON are available [24, 27-29, 34, 35, 40-42, 44, 53-55].

In 1996, Biogen initiated a trial to determine if using Avonex in individuals at high risk for developing MS could delay the development of CDMS. The study included 383 individuals at 50 clinical centers in the United States and Canada.

Individuals in this study experienced a single, isolated neurological event, like ON, suggesting demyelination, and had multiple clinically "silent" MRI lesions (and thus were at high risk for developing CDMS). The aim of the study was to determine if using Avonex early in demyelinating disease could delay the devel-opment of a second objective clinical sign of demyelinating disease (which would imply CDMS) and to determine if treatment would have an impact on MRI-detected brain lesions. The CHAMPS Study (Controlled High-Risk Subjects Avonex MS Prevention Study) was designed to take place over 5 years (including enrollment and 3 years of treatment) and included 383 individuals at 50 clinical centers in the United States and Canada.

Men and women between 18 and 50 years of age with a single clinical event within the past 2 weeks suggesting demyelination in the CNS and who had mul-tiple MRI-detected brain lesions were included. Upon enrollment, all partici-pants received a course of intravenous and oral steroid treatment, similar to the ONTT protocol. Then, subjects began weekly intramuscular injections of Avonex or placebo. Participants underwent neurological examinations and MRI brain scans every 6 months. The onset and timing of any new neurological demyelinating events were tracked, as were adverse events and side effetcs.

Avonex caused a statistically significant delay of onset of CDMS compared with the placebo-treated group (0.56, 95% confidence interval 0.38-0.81, p=0.002). In addition, over the first 3 years of the study, MRI findings showed that the treatment group had a significantly lower increase in the volume of brain lesions, as well as fewer new and enhancing lesions (p<0.001).

The CHAMPS Study indicates that once-weekly treatment with intramuscular injections of Avonex is beneficial in patients with a first presentation of demyelinating disease who are deemed to be at high risk for developing CDMS. While treatment did not prevent MS, the data suggest that the rate of development of clinically definite disease is significantly reduced. These data also indicate the benefit of obtaining MRI scans of the brain at the time of a first demyelinating event to help evaluate the possible risk for developing clinically definite disease. The study did not provide information on the longer-term benefits of early treatment with Avonex on relapse rate or disease disability [89].

In addition to CHAMPS, a similar study was organized around the same time to evaluate (22 µg) interferon β 1-a (Rebif) given subcutaneously (SC) versus placebo once weekly. This was called the Early Treatment of Multiple Sclerosis or ETOMS study [90]. The protocol for inclusion and outcome were similar to CHAMPS. Conversion from monosymptomatic events to CDMS was reduced by 24%. This is an interesting finding in that the ETOMS protocol was developed before additional clinical evidence became available that the effects of this drug given SC are dose dependent. The low dose used effectively in ETOMS for monosymptomatic events was actually shown not to be effective when used with relapsing disease (OWIMS and PRISMS Study) [91, 92]. This implies that early MS may respond in a different fashion to the relapsing-remitting type of MS.

Unfortunately, use of serial IVMP was not part of the CHAMPS or ETOMS study research design. The value of longitudinal use (perhaps monthly or quarterly) of larger-dose steroids in reducing long-term disability in very early MS is an interesting clinical research question that has yet to be answered. Regrettably, no well-designed properly powered study has appeared in the literature to document the value of longitudinally administered corticosteroid given either alone or with ABC anti-MS drugs on the reduction in disability in MS patients long term.

Discussion

Overall, the literature almost uniformly agrees that the prognosis for visual recovery in untreated ON is good. About 70% of patients recover to better than 20/20 and very few are left with poor vision. Typical cases show some improvement within 30 days [12, 13, 61, 81]. In evaluating the effect of steroids on ON or its conversion to MS, most reports have flawed design [88]. The portion of the ONTT dealing with prednisone versus placebo is a well designed study [61] (Tables 2-4). Treatment of acute monosymptomatic ON with oral prednisone in 1 mg/kg per day doses clearly confers no treatment benefit over placebo [61]. It also appears to be associated with a doubling of the recurrence rate of ON in *either eye* [61, 80], an important observation. Although this phenomena remains unexplained and controversial to some [63, 64, 83-87], it has lead directly to our recommendation that prednisone alone is of no value for treatment of ON and should be avoided in typical cases [62].

The portion of the ONTT dealing with methylprednisolone was single masked. This part of the ONTT, along with other relevant ON studies, has been used for additional recommendations. IVMP (and apparently oral methylprednisolone) speeds visual recovery, although within 1 year acuity is the same as in placebo-treated patients, according to five separate studies [56-59, 61, 82].

An important observation was that one 3-day dosage of IVMP appeared to reduce the risk of further demyelinating attacks for 2 years [73]. At the end of this time any protective effect is no longer present [80]. IVMP should be considered if the potential risks to the patient are outweighed by their requirements to have accelerated visual recovery. If MRI demonstrates three or more signal abnormalities consistent with demyelination, there appears to be a reduction of demyelinating attacks over the next 2 years when using this treatment strategy [73, 76, 80].

In patients without a diagnosis of CDMS, MRI should be considered to assess the 5-year prognosis for developing MS [19, 20, 80] and to eliminate other causes of optic neuropathy [12, 19, 23, 61]. In patients with normal MRI, a lumbar puncture can occasionally assist in determining prognosis for developing MS [21, 60]. Although forgoing the MRI, lumbar puncture and treatment are all viable practice alternatives. Given the results of the CHAMP study, MRI to help direct potential use of interferon β-1-a seems reasonable [89].

Chest X-ray, blood tests, and lumbar puncture are not necessary in evaluating patients with typical clinical features of ON [61, 78]. However, these tests may be appropriate for patients who are about to undergo glucocorticoid therapy that could complicate or unmask an unrecognized condition.

Several management issues for acute ON still lack evidence for specific recommendations. It is unclear whether treatment is beneficial in patients whose symptom duration is longer than 8 days. In addition, it is unclear whether larger doses of oral prednisone or methylprednisolone would be as beneficial as IVMP therapy. Other unanswered questions include whether a single-dose regimen of 1 g IVMP for 3 days would be as beneficial as 250 mg every 6 h for 3 days and whether oral prednisone following IVMP is needed.

The optic nerve is a highly measurable CNS white matter tract, and there are numerous methods to completely quantify in very precise detail the level of disability affecting the optic nerve. ON appears to be a forme fruste of MS based on epidemiological, HLA typing, MRI, and CSF data. This provides an excellent opportunity to use acute monosymptomatic ON as a simple and highly measurable model for therapeutic strategies in acute demyelination. The available ON literature therefore leads to some very important questions germane to the treatment of MS.

An important question to determine scientifically is if the increased ON recurrence rate associated with oral prednisone would also apply to other types of MS. As we have pointed out earlier, there is very similar epidemiology and pathophysiology between ON and MS. A June 2000 American Academy of Neurology practice parameter now defines it as a standard that lower-dose oral prednisone should not be used in ON [92]. Furthermore, we doubt that any institutional review board would or could allow an oral low-dose prednisone versus placebo trial to occur in patients with early MS based on the ONTT results in ON. Therefore, scientifically determining the actual risk versus benefit of sequential lower-dose prednisone in early MS to lower long-term disability is a mute issue.

Perhaps the most-important question to determine in long-term steroid use and MS is whether 1 g daily for 3 days of IVMP (ONTT dosages) or higher oral dosages given periodically (perhaps every 3 months or even more often) will improve long-term prognosis more than IV placebo in patients with the acute onset of MS. Further research into these and other questions raised by the acute monosymptomatic ON literature could help answer very important issues related to early MS and reduction of long-term disability.

References

1. Rizzo JF, Lessell S (1988) Risk of developing multiple sclerosis after uncomplicated optic neuritis. A long-term prospective study. Neurology 38:185-190
2. Ebers GC (1985) Optic neuritis and multiple sclerosis. Arch Neurol 42:702-704
3. Kurtzke JF (1985) Optic neuritis or multiple sclerosis. Arch Neurol 42:704-710
4. Francis DA, Compston DAS, Batchelor, McDonald WI (1987) A reassessment of the risk of multiple sclerosis developing in patients with optic neuritis after extended follow up. J Neurol Neurosurg Psychiatr 50:758-765
5. Sandberg-Wolheim M, Bynke H, Cronqvist S et al (1990) A long-term prospective study of optic neuritis: evaluation of risk factors. Ann Neurol 27:386-393
6. Perkin GD, Rose FC (1979) Optic neuritis and its differential diagnosis. Oxford, New York, pp 226-248
7. Nikoskelainen E (1975) Later course and prognosis of optic neuritis. Acta Ophthalmol (Copenh) 53:273-291
8. Hutchinson WM (1976) Acute optic neuritis and the prognosis for multiple sclerosis. J Neurol Neurosurg Psychiatr 39:283-289
9. Hely MA, McManis PG, Doran TJ, Walsh JC, McLeod JG (1986) Acute optic neuritis: a prospective study of risk factors for multiple sclerosis. J Neurol Neurosurg Psychiatr 498:1125-1130
10. Wakakura M, Ishikawa S, Oono S et al (1995) Incidence of acute idiopathic optic neuritis and its therapy in Japan. Optic Neuritis Treatment Trial Multicenter Cooperative Research Group (ONMRG). Nippon Ganka Gakkai Zasshi 99(1):93-97
11. Beck RW et al (1988) The Optic Neuritis Treatment Trial. Arch Ophthalmol 106:1051-53

12. Optic Neuritis Study Group (1991) The clinical profile of acute optic neuritis: Experience of the Optic Neuritis Treatment Trial. Arch Ophthalmol 109:1673-1678

13. Wakakura M, Minei-Higa R, Oono Shinji et al (1999) Baseline features of idiopathic optic neuritis as determined by a multi center treatment trial in Japan. Jpn J Ophthalmol 43:127-132

14. Bradley WG, Whittey WM (1967) Acute optic neuritis: its clinical features and their relation to prognosis for recovery of vision. J Neurol Neurosurg Psychiat 30:531-538

15. Rizzo JF, Lessell S (1991) Optic neuritis and ischemic optic neuropathy. Overlapping clinical profiles. Arch Ophthalmol 109:1668-1672

16. Kupersmith MJ, Nelson JI, Seiple WH, Carr RE, Weiss PA (1983) The 20/20 eye in multiple sclerosis. Neurology 33:1015-1020

17. Ashworth B, Aspinall PA, Mitchell JD (1990) Visual function in multiple sclerosis. Doc Ophthalmologica 73:209-224

18. Martinelli V, Comi G, Filippi M et al (1991) Paraclinical tests in acute-onset optic neuritis, basal data and results of a short follow up. Acta Neurol Scand 84:231-236

19. Morrissey SP, Miller DH, Kendall BE et al (1993) The significance of brain magnetic resonance imaging abnormalities at presentation with clinically isolated syndromes suggestive of multiple sclerosis. A 5-year follow-up study. Brain 116:135-146

20. Beck RW, Arrington J, Murtagh FR, Kaufman DI et al (1993) Brain MRI in acute optic neuritis experience of the optic neuritis study group. Arch Neurol 8:841-46

21. Cole SR, Beck RW, Moke PS, Kaufman DI, Tourtellotte WW, for the Optic Neuritis Study Group (1998) The predicative value of CSF oligoclonal banding for MS 5 years after optic neuritis. Neurology 51:885-887

22. Frederiksen JL, Larsson GBW, Henriksen O, Elesen J (1998) Magnetic resonance imaging of the brain in patients with acute monosymptomatic optic neuritis. Acta Neurol Scand 80:512-517

23. Jacobs L, Munschauer FE, Kaba SE (1991) Clinical and magnetic resonance imaging in optic neuritis. Neurology 41:15-19

24. Glaser GH, Merritt HH (1952) Effects of corticotrophin (ACTH) and cortisone on disorders of the nervous system. JAMA 148:898-904

25. Quinn JR, Wolfson WQ (1952) Improved results from individualized intensive hormonal treatment in certain eye diseases reported to respond poorly to ACTH or cortisone. Univ Mich Med Bull 18:1-26

26. Kazdan P, Kennedy RJ (1955) Intravenous treatment of optic neuritis. Arch Ophthalmol 53:700-701

27. Rucker CW (1956) Optic neuritis of unknown etiology. Trans Am Acad Ophthalmol Otolaryngol 60:93-96

28. Giles CL, Isaacson JD (1961) The treatment of acute optic neuritis. Arch Ophthalmol 66:52-55

29. Oksala A (1966) Cortisone therapy in fasciculitis optica. Ophthalmologica 148:13-24

30. Rawson MD, Liversedge LA, Goldfarb G, McGill BA (1966) Treatment of acute retrobulbar neuritis with corticotrophin. Lancet II:1044-1046

31. Rawson MD, Liversedge LA (1969) Treatment of retrobulbar neuritis with corticotrophin. Lancet II:222

32. Bowden AN, Bowden PMA, Friedman AI et al (1974) A trial of corticotrophin gelatin injection in acute optic neuritis. J Neurol Neurosurg Psychiatr 37:869-873

33. Gould ES, Bird AC, Leaver PK, McDonald WI (1977) Treatment of optic neuritis by retrobulbar injection of triamcinolone. BMJ 1:1485-1497

34. Mehdorn E (1990) Megadose steroid therapy in papillitis with progressive visual loss (German). Klin Monatsbl Augenheilk 197:506-513

35. van Engelen BG, Hommes OR, Pinckers A et al (1992) Improved vision after intravenous immunoglobulin in stable demyelinating optic neuritis. Ann Neurol 32(6):834-835

36. Sanders EA, Volkers AC, van der Poel JC, van Lith GH (1986) Estimation of visual function after optic neuritis; a comparison of clinical tests. Br J Ophthalmol 70:918-924

37. Fleishman JA, Beck RW, Linares OA, Klein JW (1987) Deficits in visual function after resolution of optic neuritis. Ophthalmology 94:1029-1035

38. Budning AS, Gans M, Filer R, Greenberg S (1991) Visual function after optic neuritis: a preliminary study. Can J Ophthalmol 26:18-20

39. Trauzettel-Klosinski S, Aulhorn E, Diener HD et al (1991) Effect of prednisolone on the course of optic neuritis. Results of a double-blind study (in German). Fortschr der Ophthalmol 88:490-501

40. Herishanu YO, Badarna S, Sarov B et al (1989) A possible harmful late effect of methylprednisolone therapy on a time cluster of optic neuritis. Acta Neurol Scand 80:569-574

41. Spoor TC, Rockwell DL (1988) Treatment of optic neuritis with intravenous megadose corticosteroid. A consecutive series. Ophthalmology 95:131-134

42. Farris BK, Pickard DJ (1990) Bilateral postinfectious optic neuritis and intravenous steroid therapy in children. Ophthalmology 97:339-345

43. Rollinson RD (1977) Bilateral optic neuritis in childhood. Med J Aust 9:50-51

44. Gerling J, Kommerell G (1992) Short term effect of megadose steroid therapy in optic neuritis. Klin Monatsbl Augenheilkd 201:375-380

45. Perry HD, Mallen FJ, Grodin RW, Cossari AJ (1979) Reversible blindness in optic neuritis associated with influenza vaccination. Ann Ophthalmol 11:545-550

46. Hepler RS (1976) Management of optic neuritis. Surv Ophthalmol 20:350-357

47. Dinning WJ (1976) Steroids and the eye-indications and complications. Postgrad Med J 52:634-638

48. Nano HM, Perez HA, Beraza H, Grayeb E (1970) Optic neuritis. Treatment with hydrocortisone injections. Arch Oftalmol B Aries 45:322-328

49. Huang SY, Zeng YC (1985) Clinical observations on treatment of disorders of the optic nerve by acupuncture. J Tradit Chin Med 5:187-190

50. Ershkovich IG, Gol'dfel'd-NG, Koza RI (1969) The value of glycerin and retrobulbar injections of hydrocortisone in the treatment of neuritis of the optic nerve. Oftalmol Zh 24:322-328

51. Schmidt D (1983) Treatment of optic neuritis. Bull Soc Belge Ophthalmol 208:93-96

52. Hallermann W, Haller P, Kruger C, Schiemann M, Patzold U (1983) Progress of optic neuritis with and without corticosteroid treatment. Findings in a long term investigation with static perimetry. Fortschr Ophthalmol 80:30-34

53. Toczolowski J, Lewandowska-Furmanik M, Stelmasiak Z, Wozniak D, Chmiel M (1995) Treatment of acute optic neuritis with large doses of corticosteroids. Klin Oczna 97:122-125

54. Koraszewska-Matuszewska B, Samochowiec-Donocik E, Rynkiewicz E (1995) Optic neuritis in children and adolescents. Klin Oczna 97:207-210

55. Alejandro PM, Castanon-Gonzalez JA, Miranda-Ruiz R et al (1994) Comparative treatment of acute optic neuritis with boluses of intravenous methylprednisolone or oral prednisone. Gac Med Mex 130:227-230

56. Kapoor R, Miller DH, Jones SJ et al (1998) Effects of intravenous methylprednisolone on outcome in MRI-based prognostic subgroups in acute optic neuritis. Neurology 50:230-237

57. Trauzettel-Klosinski S, Axmann D, Dienerhe HD (1993) Tubingen Study on optic neuritis treatment-a prospective, randomized and controlled trial. Clin Visual Sci 8:385-394

58. Wakakura M, Mashimo K, Oono Shinji et al (1999) Multi center clinical trial for evaluating methylprednisolone pulse treatment of idiopathic optic neuritis in Japan. Jpn J Ophthalmol 43:133-138

59. Sellebjerg F, Nielsen HS, Frederiksen JL, Olesen J (1999) A randomized, controlled trial of oral high-dose methylprednisolone in acute optic neuritis. Neurology 52:1479-1484

60. Soderstrom M, Jin Y-P, Hillert J, Link H (1998) Optic neuritis. Prognosis for multiple sclerosis from MRI, CSF, and HLA findings. Neurology 50:708-714

61. Beck RW, Cleary PA, Anderson MA et al (1992) A randomized, controlled trial of corticosteroid in the treatment of acute optic neuritis. New Eng J Med 326:581-588

62. Kaufman DI, Trobe JD, Eggenberger ER, Whitaker JN (2000) Practice parameter: the role of costicosteroids in the management of acute monosymptomatica optic neuritis. Neurology 54:2039-2044

63. Beck RW et al (1992) The Optic Neuritis Treatment Trial: implications for clinical practice. Arch Ophthalmol 110:331-332

64. Beck RW et al (1992) Corticosteroid treatment of optic neuritis: a need to change treatment practices. Neurology 42:1133-1135

65. Beck RW, Kupersmith MJ, Cleary PA et al (1993) Fellow eye abnormalities in acute unilateral optic neuritis experience of the Optic Neuritis Treatment Trial. Ophthalmology 100:691-698

66. Keltner JL, Johnson CA, Spurr JO et al (1993) Baseline visual field profile of optic neuritis. The experience of the Optic Neuritis Treatment Trial. Arch Ophthalmol 111:231-234

67. Cleary PA, Beck RW, Anderson MM et al (1993) Design, methods and conduct of the Optic Neuritis Treatment Trial. Controlled Clin Trials 14:123-142

68. Keltner JL, Johnson CA, Beck RW et al (1993) Quality control functions of the Visual Field Reading Center (VFRC) for The Optic Neuritis Treatment Trial (ONTT). Controlled Clin Trials 14:143-159

69. Beck RW, Cleary PA et al (1993) Recovery from severe visual loss in optic neuritis. Arch Ophthalmol 111:300

70. Beck RW, Diehl L, Cleary PA et al (1993) The Pelli-Robson Letter Chart: normative data for young adults. Clin Vis Sci 8:207-210

71. Chrousos GA, Kattah JC, Beck RW et al (1993) Side effects of glucocorticoid treatment: experience of the Optic Neuritis Treatment Trial. JAMA 269:2110-2112

72. Beck RW, Cleary PA et al (1993) Optic Neuritis Treatment Trial: one-year follow-up results. Arch Ophthalmol 111:773-775

73. Beck RW, Cleary PA, Trobe JD, Kaufman DI et al (1993) The effect of corticosteroid for acute optic neuritis on the subsequent development of multiple sclerosis. N Engl J Med 329:1764-1769

74. Keltner JL, Johnson CA, Spurr JO et al (1994) Visual field profile of optic neuritis: one-year follow-up in the Optic Neuritis Treatment Trial. Arch Ophthalmol 112:946-53

75. Beck RW, Cleary PA, Backlund JC et al (1994) The course of visual recovery after optic neuritis. Experience of the Optic Neuritis Treatment Trial. Ophthalmology 101:1771-1778

76. Kupersmith MJ, Kaufman D, Paty DW et al (1994) Megadose corticosteroid in multiple sclerosis. Neurology 44:1-4

77. Beck RW (1995) The Optic Neuritis Treatment Trial: three-year follow-up results. Arch Ophthalmol 113:136-137

78. Beck RW, Trobe JD (1995) The Optic Neuritis Treatment Trial: putting the results in perspective. J Neuroophthalmol 15:131-135

79. Rolak LA, Beck RW, Paty DW, Tourtellotte WW, Whitaker JN, Rudick RA, Optic Neuritis Study Group (1996) Cerebrospinal fluid in acute optic neuritis: experience of the Optic Neuritis Treatment Trial. Neurology 46:368-372

80. Optic Neuritis Study Group (1997) The 5 year risk of MS after optic neuritis. Neurology 49:1404-1413

81. Optic Neuritis Treatment Trial Manual of Operations (1990) National Technical Information Service, Springfield, Va, NTIS accession no. PB90-195728

82. Optic Neuritis Teatment Group (1997) Visual function 5 years after optic neuritis: experience of the optic neuritis treatment trial. Arch Ophthalmol 115:1545-1552

83. Goodin DS (1993) Corticosteroids and optic neuritis (letter). Neurology 43:632-633

84. Goodkin DE, Rudick RA, Kinkel R, Ransohoff RM (1993) Corticosteroids and optic neuritis (letter). Neurology 43:632-633

85. Beck RW, Optic Neuritis Study Group (1993) Corticosteroids and optic neuritis (reply). Neurology 43:633-634

86. Goodin DS (1993) Treatment of optic neuritis (letter). Neurology 43:2731

87. Beck RW, Optic Neuritis Study Group (1993) Treatment of optic neuritis (reply). Neurology 43:2731

88. Cox TA, Woolson RF (1981) Steroid treatment of optic neuritis. Arch Ophthalmol 99:338

89. Jacobs LD, Beck RW, Simon JH et al (2000) Intramuscular interferon beta-1-a therapy initiated during a first demyelinating event in multiple sclerois. N Eng J Med 343:898-904

90. Comi G, Filippi M, Barkhof F et al (2001) Effects of early interferon treatment on conversion to definite multiple sclerosis: a randomised study. Lancet 357:1576-1582

91. OWIMS Study Group (1991) Evidence of interferon B-1a dose response in relapsing remitting MS. The OWIMS Study. Neurology 53:679-686

92. Freedman MS and the Prisms Study Group (2000) Prisms 4-year results: evidence of clinical dose effect of interferon beta1-a in relapsing MS (abstract LBN.001)

Chapter 16

Antibody Mediated Demyelination*

A. Van der Goes, E.C.W. Breij, M. Kortekaas, K. Hoekstra, P.J.H. Jongen,
C.D. Dijkstra, S. Amor

Introduction

Intrathecal oligoclonal IgG antibodies (Abs) are present in more than 90% of
multiple sclerosis (MS) patients and the presence of such Abs serves as a laboratory marker supporting the diagnosis of this disease. The intrathecal IgG
fractions contain Abs with many different specificities, including myelin-specific Abs. Reports on anti-myelin Abs in cerebrospinal (CSF) and sera are controversial [1-7]. Several reports describe the presence of anti-myelin Ab in
serum and CSF, whereas others find anti-myelin Abs only in the CSF, and yet
others report that anti-myelin Abs are absent in MS patients. However, B lymphocytes specific for, and plasma cells secreting Abs to myelin basic protein
(MBP), myelin-associated glycoprotein (MAG), myelin oligodendrocyte glycoprotein (MOG), and proteolipid protein (PLP) are consistently detected in the
central nervous system (CNS) of MS patients [8-11]. Such cells are even found
in the CSF in the absence of anti-myelin Abs, suggesting that antibodies rapidly bind to target structures, such as the corresponding auto-antigens or to Fc-
receptors, and therefore become undetectable [8, 9]. In organotypic, myelinated cultures of CNS tissue, sera of MS patients promoted myelin breakdown
[12]. Similar results were obtained using rabbit anti-galactocerebroside (GalC)
sera and anti-whole myelin sera [13, 14]. Genain et al. [15] identified auto-
antibodies against MOG within acute MS lesions, where they were associated
with damaged myelin membranes, and within macrophages ingesting myelin
[15]. Lassmann et al. [16] described abundant deposition of immunoglobulins
in a subclass of active MS.

Anti-myelin Abs may not only damage myelin directly, but also contribute to
demyelination by opsonizing myelin sheats, resulting in complement deposition
and Fc receptor-mediated phagocytosis by macrophages. Although the significance of anti-myelin Abs in MS has yet to be established, in vitro studies and
studies in experimental animals suggest that auto-antibodies directed against
myelin components may play a critical pathogenic role in the disease by augmenting demyelination.

---

* This work has already been partially published in J Neuroimmunol 1999, 101:61-67

Anti-Myelin Antibodies in Experimental Allergic Encephalomyelitis

In the experimental autoimmune model of MS, experimental allergic encephalomyelitis (EAE), increased levels of Ab directed to PLP, GalC and MOG can be detected in the chronic (relapsing) demyelinating phase of the disease [17, 18]. Autoaggressive T cells initiate EAE, and many studies demonstrate that in addition to this cellular immunity, antibody responses are crucial for the development of demyelination. Injection of sera from animals with chronic EAE into the CSF of normal animals induces demyelination [19]. Whether antigen specificity plays a role in the myelin damage caused by Ab responses is not completely clear. Sera of animals with EAE only induce myelin damage in vitro following immunization with whole myelin and not with MBP alone [14]. Likewise, demyelination is only observed in animals with EAE following immunization with both MBP and GALC, and not with MBP alone [20]. Both studies indicate that for demyelination-promoting Abs, MBP may not be the major target antigen.

Other myelin antigens, particularly those present on the surface of the myelin sheath, may be important targets in antibody mediated demyelination and in the disease process. This may explain why an antibody directed to MOG, which is exclusively expressed in the CNS on the surface of myelin, augments the severity and duration of clinical signs and induces the formation of large demyelinated plaques within the CNS [21, 22]. It was shown that of a panel of anti-myelin Abs, the anti-MOG mAb Z12 induced the most severe demyelination in rats [23] and the most-severe clinical signs and demyelination in mice [17]. MOGZ12, a mouse IgG2a mAb, had the highest complement-fixing ability [23]. Treatment of mice with CVF partly abolished the MOGZ12 enhancement of the clinical signs [17], suggesting a role for complement in myelin damage [24, 25].

In summary, anti-myelin Abs can induce demyelination in vitro and do augment experimental clinical disease, but they do so to a variable extent. Understanding how such Abs exert their effects and which properties determine their disease-producing effects will be relevant to understanding the development of demyelination in MS. For this reason, we investigated the properties of a panel of anti-myelin Abs with respect to myelin phagocytosis [26].

The Role of Anti-MOG mAbs on the Phagocytosis of Myelin by Macrophages in Vitro

A panel of mAbs, raised against the minor myelin component MOG [26] was tested for ability to bind whole myelin. Myelin-binding capacities of anti-MOG clones Y1, Y4, Y6, Y7, Y9, Y10, Y11, and Z12 are depicted in Fig. 1. The strongest binding of mAb with myelin was observed with the mAb MOGZ12, while the mAb MOG Y1, MOGY4, MOGY10, and MOGY11 bound to mice myelin to a somewhat lesser extent. MOGY7 and MOGY9 showed only weak binding and MOGY6 was not able to bind myelin. The differences in binding were not related to the isotype of the Ab.

Subsequently, phagocytosis of Ab-treated myelin by murine macrophages was determined in vitro using a quantitative flow cytometric assay. Purified murine

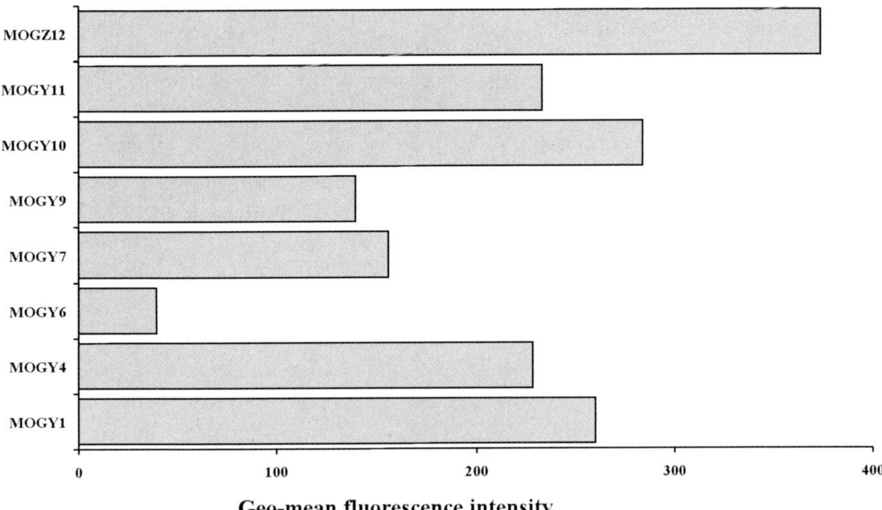

Fig. 1. Incubation of mouse myelin with monoclonal antibody (mAb) against myelin oligodendrocyte glycoprotein (*MOG*). The binding is visualized by incubating the mAb-myelin with fluorescent-labeled conjugates. The fluorescence intensity of the myelin was measured using FACScan flow cytometry. Both methods and data have been published previously [26]. The data are presented as the geo-mean of fluorescence of one representative experiment ($n=4$)

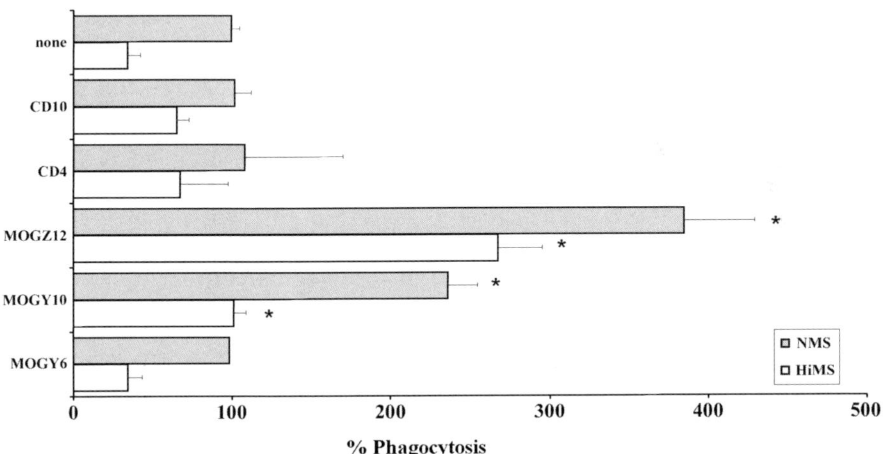

Fig. 2. Phagocytosis of mouse myelin, which was pre-incubated with anti-MOG mAb, by J774.2 cells. Both methods and data have been published previously [26]. Data are presented as the mean percentage of binding and uptake of the fluorescent myelin±SEM of five experiments. $^*p \leq 0.05$

myelin labeled with DiI was incubated with anti-MOG mAb. Compared with untreated myelin, pretreatment with myelin-specific mAbs modified the degree of phagocytosis (Fig. 2). The efficiency of myelin opsonization was related to the isotype of antibody, the epitope recognized, and the ability of the mAbs to fix complement. The greatest degree of opsonization of myelin was observed with the mAb MOG Z12 that has previously been shown to enhance clinical signs and demyelination in EAE. In contrast to MOGZ12, an IgG2a mAb, the opsonizing effect of MOGY10 (IgG1) was less. This is in agreement with the observation that MOG Y10 did not enhance clinical disease or demyelination in the mouse EAE model. The different effects of the Abs may be dependent on the affinity for myelin and the ability of these mAbs to fix complement. Indeed Piddlesden et al. [23] demonstrated that while all the anti-MOG mAbs are capable of fixing complement, MOGZ12 is able to fix complement much more efficiently than any of the IgG1 mAbs. Our data reveal that mAbs that are most effective in promoting EAE show the highest rate of binding to myelin and the greatest enhancement of myelin phagocytosis in vitro [26].

Because of the ability of Fcγ receptors (FcγR) to induce inflammation upon Ab binding, these receptors may be involved in Ab-mediated demyelination. Furthermore, given the ability of Abs to fix complement, complement receptors may also play a role in Ab-mediated demyelination. Depending on the involvement of subclasses of complement receptor and FcγR in Ab-mediated demyelination, the disease outcome may differ. Thus, the determination of the subclasses of complement and FcγR that are involved in Ab-mediated demyelination should be performed. Interestingly, studies in FcγR knockout mice suggest an important role for both stimulatory and inhibitory Fcγ receptors in EAE [27, 28].

Anti-Myelin Auto-Abs in CSF of MS Patients

The use of the in vitro myelin phagocytosis assay offers possibilities for the analysis of the opsonizing capacities of anti-myelin auto-Abs in CSF of MS patients. Such studies may give an indication as to the extent of Ab-mediated demyelination in MS patients, and thus provide a helpful tool to classify subtypes of MS. Such classification could be relevant for the development of specific therapeutic strategies for this heterogeneous disease.

In a pilot study we have used fluorescence-activated cell sorting (FACS) analysis to investigate whether CSF samples of MS patients contain anti-myelin auto-Abs (Fig. 3). Our results demonstrate that FACS analysis of human myelin incubated with CSF and a fluorescent conjugate can be used to detect anti-myelin auto-Abs in the CSF of MS patients. The advantage of this method above those that test the presence of Abs against selected myelin proteins (e.g. MBP, MAG, MOG, and PLP) is that Abs against unknown or unexpected myelin antigens may also be detected. By testing anti-myelin-positive CSF samples in a phagocytosis assay it can be determined whether the anti-myelin auto-Abs that are present in the CSF of MS patients are also capable of increasing myelin phagocytosis. Such functional analysis of large numbers of CSF samples and correlation with clinical disease type will reveal implications for the clinical situation.

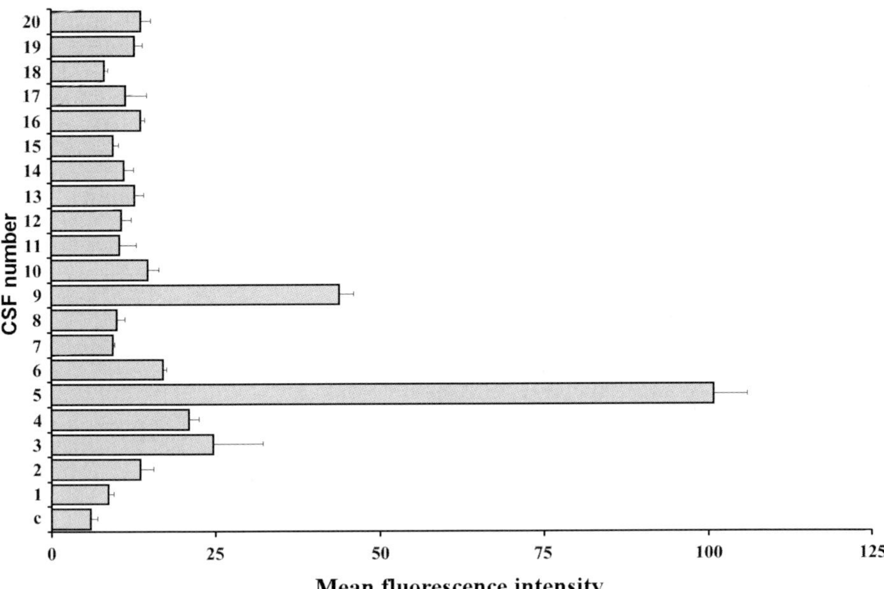

Fig. 3. Cerebrospinal fluid (*CSF*) of 10 multiple sclerosis patients (CSF 1 to CSF 10) and 10 control patients (CSF 11 to CSF 20) were used. Myelin isolated from normal human white matter was incubated with CSF. After an overnight incubation at 4°C, the non-bound Abs were washed away and the myelin was incubated with fluorescent-labeled conjugate (goat anti-humanIgG-phycoerythrin). After an incubation of 1 h, the non-bound conjugate was washed away and the fluorescence intensity of the myelin was measured using a FACScan flow cytometer. The data are presented as the geo-mean of fluorescence of one representative experiment (*n*=3). The CSF showed varying degrees of binding. The maximum binding was observed with CSF 5 and CSF 9, while CSF 3, 4, and 6 bound to human myelin to a lesser extent. In contrast, CSF 1, 2, 7, 8, and 10 showed a binding to myelin which was comparable to the 10 control CSF samples (CSF 11 to CSF 20)

Conclusions and Perspectives

This short review on the role of Abs in demyelination shows that there are indications that Abs may influence the course of the disease. Tools are available to detect anti-myelin Abs in CSF or blood of MS patients and to estimate the capacity of these antibodies to enhance demyelination in vitro. The question arises whether the presence of demyelination-promoting Abs in CSF or serum of MS patients can be correlated with specific clinical features. Further research should be performed to investigate whether the presence of such Abs could serve as a tool to diagnose clinical subtypes of MS. This may be relevant to the development of specific therapeutic strategies for this heterogeneous disease. These issues are currently being addressed in our department.

Acknowledgements. This work was supported financially by the Dutch foundation "Vrienden MS Research", project MS 95-202 and the Multiple Sclerosis Society of Great Britain and Northern Ireland. We would like to thank Dr. K.J.B. Lamers (Department of Neurology, Academic Hospital Nijmegen, The Netherlands) and Dr. P.J.H. Jongen (MS Centre Nijmegen, The Netherlands) for providing us with the CSF samples.

References

1. Möller JR et al (1989) Antibodies to myelin-associated glycoprotein (MAG) in the cerebrospinal fluid of multiple sclerosis patients. J Neuroimmunol 22:55-61
2. Cruz M et al (1987) Immunoblot detection of oligoclonal anti-myelin basic protein IgG antibodies in cerebrospinal fluid in multiple sclerosis. Neurology 37:1515-1519
3. Henneberg A et al (1991) Antibodies to brain tissue in sera of patients with chronic progressive multiple sclerosis. J Neuroimmunol 34:223-227
4. Bernard CCA et al (1981) Antibody to myelin basic protein in extracts of multiple sclerosis brain. Immunology 43:447-457
5. Ryberg B, Jacque C (1986) Are anti-brain antibodies in multiple sclerosis directed to myelin basic protein. Acta Neurol Scand 73:247-252
6. Wajgt A, Górny M (1983) CSF antibodies to myelin basic protein and to myelin-associated glycoprotein in multiple sclerosis. Evidence of the intrathecal production of antibodies. Acta Neurol Scand 68:337-343
7. Xiao BX et al (1991) Antibodies to myelin-oligodendrocyte glycoprotein in cerebrospinal fluid from patients with multiple sclerosis and controls. J Neuroimmunol 31:91-96
8. Sun JB et al (1991) T and B cell responses to myelin-oligodendrocye glycoprotein in multiple sclerosis. J Immunol 146:1490-1495
9. Sun JB et al (1991) Autoreactive T and B cells responding to myelin proteolipid in multiple sclerosis and controls. Eur J Immunol 21:1461-1468
10. Baig S et al (1991) Multiple sclerosis: cells secreting antibodies against myelin-associated glycoprotein are present in cerebrospinal fluid. Scand J Immunol 33:73-79
11. Link H et al (1990) Persistent anti-myelin basic protein IgG antibody response in multiple sclerosis cerebrospinal fluid. J Neuroimmunol 28:237-248
12. Raine CS et al (1973) Multiple sclerosis: serum-induced demyelination in vitro. J Neurol Sci 20:127-148
13. Seil FJ (1968) The in vitro demyelinating activity of sera from guinea pigs sensitized with while CNS and with purified encephalitogen. Exp Neurol 22:545-555
14. Raine CS et al (1981) Demyelination in vitro: absorption studies demonstrate that galactocerebroside is a major target. J Neurolog Sci 52:117-131
15. Genain CP et al (1999) Identification of autoantibodies with myelin damage in multiple sclerosis. Nat Med 5:170-175
16. Lassmann H et al (2001) Heterogeneity of multiple sclerosis pathogenesis: implications for diagnosis and therapy. Trends Mol Med 7:115-121
17. Morris MM et al (1998) Antibodies to myelin components modulate experimental allergic encephalomyelitis in Biozzi ABH (H-2A^{g7}) mice. Biochem Soc Trans 25:168S-173S
18. Linington C, Lassmann H (1987) Antibody responses in chronic relapsing experimental allergic encephalomyelitis: correlation of serum demyelinating activity with antibody titre to the myelin/oligodendrocyte glycoprotein (MOG). J Neuroimmunol 17:61-69

19. Lassmann H et al (1981) In vivo effect of sera from animals with chronic relapsing experimental allergic encephalomyelitis on central and peripheral myelin. Acta Neuropathol (Berl) 55:297-306
20. Moore GRW et al (1984) Experimental autoimmune encephalomyelitis: augmentation of demyelination by different myelin lipids. Lab Invest 51:416-424
21. Linington C et al (1988) Augmentation of demyelination in rat acute allergic encephalomyelitis by circulating mouse monoclonal antibodies directed against a myelin/ologodendrocyte glycoprotein. Am J Pathol 130:443-454
22. Schluesner HJ et al (1987) A monoclonal antibody against a myelin ologodendrocyte glycoprotein induces relapses and demyelination in central nervous system autoimmune disease. J Immunol 139:4016-4021
23. Piddlesden SJ et al (1993) The demyelinating potential of antibodies to myelin oligodendrocyte glycoprotein is related to their ability to fix complement. Am J Pathol 143:555-564
24. Piddlesden SJ et al (1991) Antibody-mediated demyelination in experimental allergic encephalomyelitis is independent of complement membrane attack complex formation. Exp Immunol 83:245-250
25. Piddlesden SJ et al (1994) Soluble recombinant complement receptor 1 inhibits inflammation and demyelination in antibody-mediated demyelinating experimental allergic encephalomyelitis. J Immunol 152:5477-5484
26. Van der Goes A et al (1999) The role of anti-myelin (auto)-antibodies in the phagocytosis of myelin by macrophages. J Neuroimmunol 101:61-67
27. Abdul-Majid K et al (2002) Fc Receptors are critical for autoimmune inflammatory damage to the central nervous system in experimental autoimmune encephalomyelitis. Scand J Immunol 55:70-81
28. Lock C (2002) Gene-microarray analysis of multiple sclerosis lesions yields new targets validated in autoimmune encephalomyelitis. Nat Med 8:500-508

Anti-MOG Antibodies as Early Predictors for Conversion to Relapsing-Remitting Disease Course in Patients Suggestive of Multiple Sclerosis

T. BERGER, P. RUBNER, R. EGG, E. DILITZ, D. STADLBAUER, F. DEISENHAMMER, C. LININGTON, M. REINDL

Introduction

Multiple sclerosis (MS) is the most common neurological disease in young adults, with the potential for subsequent chronic functional impairment and disability. MS exhibits not only heterogeneous clinical manifestations and disease courses but also heterogeneous neuropathological features. Recently, different neuropathological subtypes were defined, one characterized by features of antibody mediated immunopathogenesis [1]. A potential target antigen for autoreactive antibodies might be the central nervous system (CNS) specific myelin oligodendrocyte glycoprotein (MOG), which is exclusively localized on the surface of myelin sheaths and oligodendrocytes.

Most recently we demonstrated that a substantial subgroup of MS patients mounts a persistent autoantibody response to the extracellular immunoglobulin-domain of MOG in cerebrospinal fluid (CSF) and serum [2]. These anti-MOG antibodies are present early in MS, whereas frequencies of antibodies against other myelin antigens, e.g., myelin basic protein (MBP), are low in early MS and increase during disease progression in relapsing-remitting and chronic progressive MS, suggesting that anti-MBP antibodies accumulate over time.

In general, the individual MS course is unpredictable at onset and requires dissemination in time as well as observation/monitoring over a long period. In patients with the very first symptoms of multiple sclerosis (MSR0), the uncertainty of prediction and prognosis causes uncertainty regarding the timing of treatment initiation. Although results of early treatment trials (ETOMS, CHAMPS) will be presented soon, initiation of immunomodulatory therapies requires a second MS relapse presently.

Therefore we were interested whether the presence of anti-MOG antibodies in patients with suspected MS predicts the disease course, namely the time interval to the second disease relapse and therefore conversion to definite relapsing-remitting MS.

Patients and Methods

Inclusion Criteria
– Patients with first acute neurological symptoms and signs suggestive of MS

- Positive magnetic resonance imaging (MRI) scan characterized by typical disseminated white matter lesions
- Positive oligoclonal bands in CSF
- Follow-up period of clinical monitoring for acute relapses ≥12 months

Exclusion Criteria

- Patients with a previous history of *any kind* of neurological symptoms or signs
- Patients with monotopic clinical symptoms or MRI lesions, e.g., optic neuritis or transverse myelitis without disseminated white matter lesions in MRI or positive oligoclonal bands
- Patients with clinical, laboratory, MRI, or CSF features suggestive for any other differential diagnosis than MS
- Patients receiving any immunosuppressive or immunomodulatory treatment during either diagnostic serum/CSF sampling at disease onset (e.g., high-dose methylprednisolone) or clinical follow-up period until the second MS relapse
- Follow-up period of clinical monitoring for acute relapses < 12 months
- Patients with primary progressive MS (defined at month 12)

Ninety-seven patients were enrolled in this study. Neurological examinations, including repeated rigorous interviews upon any event suggestive for an acute relapse or disease progression, were performed every 3-6 months. Twenty-four patients had to be excluded because they did not meet the criteria of at least 12 months of clinical follow-up on 29 February 2000. Anti-MOG and anti-MBP antibodies were measured in our laboratory as described previously [2].

For statistical analysis (means, standard deviations) and significance of group differences (Mann-Whitney U tests, *t*-tests) the SPSS statistical analysis program (SPSS) was used. *P*-values <0.05 were considered as statistically significant.

Results

Results are shown in Table 1 and Fig. 1.

Table 1. Mean duration (months) from first to second multiple sclerosis relapse in patients with or without antibodies against myelin oligoderdrocyte glycoprotein (*MOG*) and myelin basic (*MBP*)

Antibodies	Patients (*n*=73)	Sex (F:M)	Age at disease onset (years)	Months to 2nd relapse	Mean (months)	S D (months)
MOG–/MBP–	21 (29%)	1.6:1	32.8	606	28.9*, **	10.7
MOG+/MBP–	39 (53%)	2.9:1	31.1	420	10.7*	7.6
MOG+/MBP+	13 (18%)	3.3:1	29.3	95	7.3**	4.8

* *p*<0.001, ** *p*<0.001

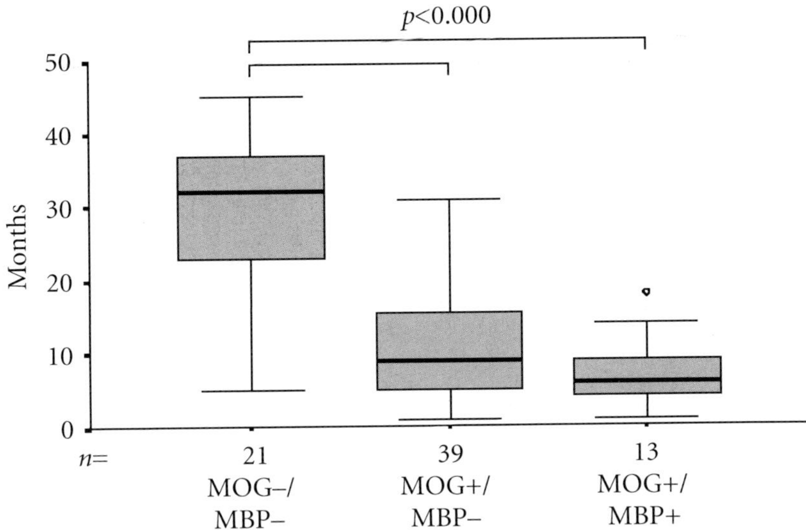

Fig. 1. Time (months) from first to second multiple sclerosis relapse in patients with or without antibodies against myelin oligodendrocyte glycoprotein (*MOG*) and myelin basic protein (*MBP*). Lines within each box represent median values, the extremes of each box indicate the 25th and 75th percentiles, the error bars show the 10th and 90th percentiles and the *circles* indicate the outliers

Discussion

We demonstrated for the first time that in MSR0 patients the detection of antibodies against MOG and MBP predicts conversion to definite relapsing-remitting MS. MSR0 patients are a very special population of suggested MS patients, where neurological symptoms and signs, MRI examinations, and CSF investigations suggest the first attack of MS. However, in general, no clinical, radiological, or immunological parameter allows prediction of an anticipated relapsing-remitting disease course. In addition, definite diagnosis and therefore treatment initiation, requires observation over time, namely occurrence of a second acute MS relapse.

Our study demonstrates that MSR0 patients with antibodies against MOG and MOG/MBP, respectively, have a high risk of developing a second acute relapse within 7-10 months. Thus, our study further supports the concept that a subgroup of patients should receive early treatment to prevent definite conversion to relapsing-remitting MS at the earliest possible time.

Acknowledgements. This study was supported by a research grant from the Austrian Federal Ministery of Science.

References

1. Luccinetti CF, Brück W, Rodriguez M, Lassmann H (1996) Distinct patterns of multiple sclerosis pathology indicates heterogeneity in pathogenesis. Brain Pathol 6:259-274
2. Reindl M, Linington C, Brehm U, Egg R, Dilitz E, Deisenhammer F, Berger T (1999) Antibodies against the myelin oligodendrocyte glycoprotein and the myelin basic protein in multiple sclerosis and other neurological diseases: a comparative study. Brain 122:2047-2056

Chapter 18

Sunlight, Vitamin D, and Multiple Sclerosis

C.E. Hayes

Environmental Risk Factors and Multiple Sclerosis

The biological mechanisms leading to multiple sclerosis (MS) are uncertain, but both genetic and environmental factors contribute to establishment and progression of the disease [1]. Compared with unrelated individuals, biological first-degree relatives of MS patients show a 20- to 40-fold increased risk of disease, and this increased risk is attributable to genetic factors, rather than a transmissible agent [2]. However, 70% of monozygotic twin pairs are discordant for MS, indicating that inheriting MS susceptibility genes is not sufficient for disease development [3]. Thus, MS development requires exposure to one or more environmental risk factors. This suggests that MS may be preventable if these risk factors can be identified and avoided.

MS prevalence shows a striking geographic distribution that strongly suggests an environmental risk factor. The disease prevalence increases with increasing latitude in both hemispheres, from a low of 1-2 cases per 10^5 population near the equator, to a high of >200 cases per 10^5 population at latitudes >50° [4]. Of all the latitude-linked variables examined, the most-significant inverse correlation with MS prevalence was average annual sunshine ($r = -0,80$), implying that sunlight might be protective in MS [4]. A recent large and thorough epidemiological study found that individuals exposed to the highest levels of residential and occupational sunlight had a significantly lower risk of mortality from MS (odds ratio 0.24) and higher risk of mortality from melanoma (odds ratio 1.38) than those with the least sunlight exposure [5].

Separating genetic and environmental influences is difficult in epidemiological studies. However, studies involving genetically similar populations have reinforced the possibility that sunlight may be protective in MS. For example, in the United States, the lower mortality risk from MS among individuals exposed to residential and occupational sunlight was independent of country of origin, age, sex, race, or socioeconomic status [5]. In Switzerland, low-altitude districts (≤1,000 m) had high MS rates, whereas high-altitude districts (≥2,000 m) had low MS rates, despite the relative genetic similarity of the two populations [6]. These results may reflect increased solar radiation intensity with increasing altitude, and also the fact that particles in the polluted air that collects in the industrial valleys filter out the ultraviolet (UV) portion of the spectrum.

Importantly, immigrants displayed the MS risk of their new homeland, reinforcing the conclusion that the latitude gradient of MS risk reflects environmental rather than genetic variables [7]. For example, Irish immigrants to Hobart, Australia (42.8°S) had an MS prevalence about five-fold higher than Irish immigrants to Queensland, Australia (25.1°S), similar to native-born Australians, regardless of age at migration [8]. These conclusions are consistent with a large number of previous migration studies [7].

Together, these geographic, climatological, and epidemiological studies suggest that low exposure to sunlight may be a significant environmental risk factor for MS, and further, that sunlight may be beneficial in those with a genetic risk of MS at all ages, not just in childhood and early adulthood. The strong inverse correlation between MS prevalence and sunlight exposure led to the hypothesis that vitamin D may be a natural inhibitor of MS [9-11].

Sunlight, Vitamin D, and MS

The vitamin D endocrine system is exquisitely responsive to sunlight. Vitamin D is sometimes called the sunshine vitamin, but in fact, it is the precursor of a secosteroid hormone, not a "vital amine" as the early twentieth century nomenclature might suggest [12]. All vertebrates, including humans, obtain their vitamin D requirement mainly from a chemical reaction in skin that is exposed to sunlight [13]. It is exceptionally difficult to obtain adequate vitamin D solely from the diet [12]. Sunlight catalyzes previtamin D_3 synthesis in skin [14]. The energy of the UV-B photons that penetrate the epidermis is absorbed by 7-dehydrocholesterol, rupturing the 9-10 carbon-carbon bond, and yielding an unstable intermediate, previtamin D_3. This compound spontaneously isomerizes to vitamin D_3. Vitamin D_3 is transported from the skin to the liver bound to the serum vitamin D binding protein. In hepatocytes, C-25 hydroxylation produces the major circulating form of vitamin D, 25-hydroxyvitamin D_3 [25-(OH)-D_3]. In the kidney, a highly regulated C-1 hydroxylation produces a biologically active hormone, 1,25-dihydroxyvitamin D_3 [1,25-$(OH)_2$-D_3] [15, 16].

Latitude and season affect the intensity of solar radiation reaching the earth's surface, and therefore the rate of vitamin D synthesis [17]. In winter and at high latitudes, sunlight strikes the earth at an oblique angle, and filters through a great stratospheric distance that decreases the UV-B radiation. In Boston, Massachusetts (42°N), there was insufficient sunlight to support vitamin D synthesis from November through February. Further north in Edmonton, Canada (52°N), vitamin D synthesis stopped from October through March. In Los Angeles, California (34°N), vitamin D synthesis occurred year round. Consequently, people living at northerly or southerly latitudes, who do not eat vitamin D-rich foods or supplements, are at a significant risk of becoming vitamin D deficient during the winter.

Genetic and Biological Evidence Correlating Vitamin D and MS Inhibition

Evidence consistent with the hypothesis that vitamin D may be a natural inhibitor of MS also derives from genetic studies, human biological investigations, and animal experiments. The secosteroid hormone mediates its activities primarily through a nuclear vitamin D hormone receptor (VDR). The VDR regulates the transcription of particular genes, mainly through a vitamin D-responsive element in the promoter region [18, 19]. We hypothesized that mutations in the genes involved in vitamin D metabolism and function might be associated with MS susceptibility, but we found no correlation between MS and genetic markers at the Chromosome (Chr) 12q14 *VDR* locus, the Chr 12q13 gene encoding the 25-hydroxyvitamin D_3 1-α-hydroxylase, or the Chr 4q12 *Gc* locus encoding the vitamin D binding protein in Canadian families [20]. In Iceland, the *Gc-1f* allele was associated with MS [21]. Moreover, in Japan, the *VDR* gene *b* allele (presence of a *Bsm* I restriction endonuclease site) was over-represented in MS patients ($p=0.0138$) [22]. This result was confirmed using a second *VDR* genetic marker, and an association between this *VDR* allele and the *HLA DPB1*0501* allele was observed in the MS patients [23]. This association is significant, in that the *HLA DP* gene may be involved in autoantigen presentation to T lymphocytes, and the *VDR* gene may regulate T cell responsiveness to autoantigens [24].

Nutritional studies have provided some data consistent with the vitamin D and MS hypothesis. Fish oil is a rich vitamin D source, and there is limited evidence that diets rich in fish may lower the incidence and/or severity of MS. Coastal Norway had lower MS prevalence rates than inland Norway [25]. The coastal Norwegians consumed about 1,300 IU of vitamin D3 daily, about three-fold higher than individuals living inland [9]. Furthermore, in a small, uncontrolled, non-blinded clinical trial, MS patients ingesting cod liver oil (20 g/day, 5,000 IU/day of vitamin D), along with calcium and magnesium supplements, had lower exacerbation rates [26]. Another uncontrolled, non-blinded trial reported that MS patients counseled to consume fish (8 times/day) and fish oil (0.9 g/day) had fewer exacerbations and lower disability scores than prior to the diet change [27]. Other nutritional changes were made, and serum vitamin D measurements were not recorded, so the interpretation of these results is uncertain. Despite the methodological shortcomings in these two small fish oil trials, when the results are taken in the context of the other evidence, they contribute to the theory that vitamin D may be a natural inhibitor of MS.

Additional evidence comes from the data indicating that MS patients exhibit long-term vitamin D deficiency, as characterized by low bone mass and high fracture rates. The best indicator of near-term vitamin D nutrition is serum 25-(OH)-D_3, which was less than adequate (<50 nmol/l) in 69% of MS patients [28, 29]. Compared with their age- and gender-matched healthy peers, the MS patients had significantly reduced bone mass, which is indicative of long-term vitamin D malnutrition [28]. Finally, MS patients lost bone mass at a three- to seven-fold higher rate and experienced fractures at a ten-fold higher rate than their peers [28]. These findings indicate that significant vitamin D deficiency of some duration exists in most MS patients.

Critically important evidence for a connection between sunlight, vitamin D, and MS comes from studies on seasonal variations in the disease. Disease onset and exacerbations frequently occurred in the spring [30-33]. Studies on the seasonal fluctuations of gadolinium-enhancing, magnetic resonance imaging (MRI) lesions in MS patients [34] and serum 25-(OH)D$_3$ levels [35] found that brain lesion frequency peaked about 2 months after the nadir of serum 25-(OH)D$_3$ levels, while the nadir of brain lesion frequency occurred about 2 months after serum 25-(OH)D$_3$ levels peaked. The temporal correlation between MS severity and serum 25-(OH)D3 levels points to a possible cause and effect relationship between lack of vitamin D and increased MS severity. It will be important to measure serum 25-(OH)-D$_3$ levels in MS patients to substantiate the evidence correlating MS disease activity with seasonal variations in vitamin D synthesis.

We and others have provided extensive evidence that the biologically active hormone 1,25-(OH)$_2$D$_3$ inhibits experimental autoimmune encephalomyelitis (EAE), a model of MS. Immunizing mice with spinal cord homogenate induced a progressively paralytic autoimmune disease, EAE, with strong similarities to MS [36]. In this model, 1,25-(OH)$_2$D$_3$ treatment completely blocked EAE induction and progression of established EAE [37]. The lower the dietary calcium level, the higher the 1,25-(OH)$_2$-D$_3$ dose needed to completely prevent EAE symptoms, suggesting that adequate dietary calcium is important for EAE inhibition [38]. Others reported partial inhibition of EAE morbidity and mortality [39]. Furthermore, we showed that mice with severe acute EAE recovered from paralysis within a few days of 1,25-(OH)$_2$D$_3$ treatment, and the recovery correlated with a rapid depletion of inflammatory macrophages from the central nervous system (CNS) [40]. Together these experiments indicate that 1,25-(OH)$_2$D$_3$ is a profoundly important EAE inhibitor.

The mechanism whereby 1,25-(OH)$_2$-D$_3$ inhibits EAE is not known. Myeloid lineage cells and activated T lymphocytes possess this VDR [41, 42]. In particular, the CD4$^+$ T helper type-1 (Th1) and type-2 (Th2) [24] and CD8$^+$ T cells [43] express VDR mRNA, suggesting that they may be targets of the hormone immune system regulation. Several investigators have shown that 1,25-(OH)$_2$D$_3$ is a potent and specific inhibitor of activated Th1 cells in vitro [42, 44-48]. Others have shown that 1,25-(OH)$_2$D$_3$ decreased interleukin-12 (IL-12) production in vitro [49, 50], and inhibited dendritic cell (DC) maturation, activation, and antigen-presenting cell function in vitro [51-53]. Since DC producing IL-12 are strong stimulators of Th1 differentiation [54], and Th1 cells are encephalitogenic in EAE [55], one possible mechanism for 1,25-(OH)$_2$D$_3$ inhibition of EAE induction would be for the hormone to inhibit DC functions, thereby diminishing Th1 cell differentiation and/or function.

We tested the hypothesis that $1,25\text{-}(OH)_2D_3$ might inhibit Th1 cell differentiation and/or Th1 cell function in vivo [24]. The studies used T lymphocytes from T cell receptor- (TCR-) transgenic mice [56], so the T cells specific for myelin basic protein peptide (MBP), here termed TCR1 T cells, could be recovered and analyzed. The effects of $1,25\text{-}(OH)_2D_3$ treatment on TCR1 T cell differentiation and function were examined in cell transfer experiments in vivo and in cell culture experiments in vitro. The $1,25\text{-}(OH)_2D_3$ treatment inhibited EAE induction in mice that received the TCR1 cells and a priming dose of peptide. However, it did not inhibit Th1 cell development or function in the peripheral lymph nodes, or promote Th2 cell development or function, or stimulate TCR1 T cell deletion. Remarkably, in the $1,25\text{-}(OH)_2D_3$-treated mice, there were TCR1 T cells in the CNS but they were not activated, whereas the mock-treated mice had activated, MBP-responsive TCR1 T cells in the CNS, correlating with their EAE disease symptoms. When the same experiment was performed in mice that were *Rag-1* deficient, the $1,25\text{-}(OH)_2D_3$ treatment did not inhibit EAE induction. This important result ruled out a direct effect of the hormone on antigen-presenting cell function, or on the autoreactive T cells to shift them towards a Th2 phenotype [57, 58], and instead, signaled a requirement for *Rag-1*-dependent cells in EAE inhibition. This new evidence suggests that the $1,25\text{-}(OH)_2D_3$ treatment may inhibit EAE by enhancing a *Rag-1*-dependent cell that limits activation of neural antigen-specific T cells in the CNS.

Several mechanisms prevent activation of injurious, neural antigen-specific T cells in the CNS, and one of them is active suppression. Despite their excessive numbers of neural antigen-specific T cells, the TCR1 mice do not spontaneously develop EAE unless they are *Rag-1*-null [59, 60]. Further gene knock-out experiments demonstrated that the *Rag-1*-dependent suppressor cells were $TCR\alpha\beta$ $CD4^+$ T cells. Moreover, suppression of neural antigen-reactive T cell activation occurred in the CNS, but not in the peripheral lymph nodes, so this tolerance mechanism operates in situ, not systemically [61]. Additional experiments will be required to determine whether neural antigen-specific suppressor cells are present in the CNS of the disease-free, $1,25\text{-}(OH)_2D_3$-treated mice as our data imply [24], and these experiments are in progress. However, we hypothesize that the $1,25\text{-}(OH)_2D_3$ is augmenting the development and/or function of regulatory T cells that maintain self tolerance in the periphery. If this hypothesis is correct, then lack of sufficient vitamin D to support $1,25\text{-}(OH)_2D_3$ biosynthesis could be an environmental risk factor for a large number of autoimmune disorders.

Vitamin D Inhibition of Type I Diabetes Mellitus and Other Autoimmune Diseases

It is important to note that vitamin D and the hormone $1,25\text{-}(OH)_2\text{-}D_3$ have been implicated in the inhibition of other human autoimmune diseases and many mouse autoimmune disease models. Type I (insulin-dependent) diabetes (IDDM) prevalence increases with increasing latitude, and there is an inverse correlation between incidence and mean monthly sunshine hours [62-67]. Also, in Japanese families, the VDR gene *b* allele was implicated in susceptibility to IDDM in Indian Asians [68]. Importantly, a recent study correlated vitamin D supplementation in early childhood with significantly reduced risk for IDDM [69]. Moreover, $1,25\text{-}(OH)_2\text{-}D_3$ prevented insulitis and diabetes in the non-obese diabetic mouse [70]. Together, these studies provide evidence for a protective role of vitamin D in IDDM.

There may also be a protective role of vitamin D in inflammatory bowel diseases (IBD) such as Crohn's disease and ulcerative colitis. IBD shows the same latitude gradient as MS and IDDM [71-74]. Moreover, high IBD mortality is associated with indoor work, while low IBD mortality is associated with outdoor occupations [75-77]. In addition, fish oil consumption lessened IBD symptoms [78-80]. Finally, $1,25\text{-}(OH)_2\text{-}D_3$ inhibited the induction of dextran sodium sulfate-induced colitis in mice and reduced the disease severity in the chronic dextran sodium sulfate colitis model (C.E. Hayes and F.E. Nashold, unpublished).

There is also evidence from other animal models of autoimmune disease. $1,25\text{-}(OH)_2\text{-}D_3$ inhibited experimental autoimmune thyroiditis [81], experimental murine lupus [82], and both collagen-induced arthritis and Lyme arthritis [83]. Underlying these diverse observations in so many autoimmune diseases may be a fundamental biological requirement for vitamin D to sustain immunological health, in particular to maintain self tolerance.

Vitamin D Nutrition and Immunological Self Tolerance

If the vitamin D endocrine system is essential to maintain self tolerance, a crucial unanswered question is what level of vitamin D may be needed. Vitamin D has important physiological roles beyond its skeletal functions. For example, vitamin D insufficiency is associated with hypertension, and cancers of the breast, colon, and prostate [12, 84]. There is an emerging view that the amount of the secosteroid required for the non-skeletal functions may be higher than the amount required to maintain bone health [12, 84]. The serum $25\text{-}(OH)\text{-}D_3$ level is the most-reliable indicator of near-term vitamin D nutrition. The currently accepted threshold for adequate vitamin D nutrition with respect to bone health is 50 nmol/l [85]. Hyperparathyroidism accompanies poor vitamin D nutrition, and parathyroid hormone levels did not decline to a plateau until serum $25\text{-}(OH)\text{-}D_3$ levels rose to about 60-70 nmol/l [85, 86]. In the seasonal study of active MS lesions, the nadir occurred when serum $25\ (OH)\text{-}D_3$ levels in the control subjects reached about 65 nmol/l [35]. Furthermore, the circulating $25\text{-}(OH)\text{-}D_3$ levels are between 105 and 163 nmol/l in sunny environments where MS prevalence is lowest [87]. Studies explicitly measuring serum 25-

(OH)-D$_3$ levels and correlating these with MS prevalence and MS disease activity are needed to provide guidance on optimal 25-(OH)-D$_3$ levels from the perspective of MS. In the absence of explicit information, the studies cited above indicate the optimal serum 25-(OH)-D$_3$ level to support self tolerance might be between 70 and 100 nmol/l.

If vitamin D is a natural inhibitor of MS, it would be reasonable to provide supplemental vitamin D to individuals who are at risk for MS. However, there has been uncertainty regarding how much vitamin D may be needed to maintain the estimated optimal serum 25-(OH)-D$_3$ level of 70 to 100 nmol/l. The National Academy of Sciences of the United States and The Food and Nutrition Board of the Institute of Medicine in the United States determined that an adequate intake of vitamin D is 200 IU/day (5 µg/day) for individuals aged 19-50 years [88]. This intake prevents rickets, a metabolic bone disease, but it does not prevent secondary hyperparathyroidism and osteoporosis in adults [85, 88]. There are other indications that this intake is considerably too low. Of individuals taking multivitamins (400 IU/day of vitamin D), 46% had low serum 25-(OH)-D$_3$ levels [89]. Even an intake of 600 IU/day was not enough to prevent vitamin D insufficiency in veiled ethnic Danish Moslems [90] or submariners [91] who were sunlight deprived.

The emerging view is that 800-1,000 IU/day may be required to achieve 25-(OH)-D$_3$ levels in the 50 nmol/l range if sun exposure is limited [89, 90, 92]. To maintain a serum 25-(OH)-D$_3$ level of approximately 100 nmol/l, similar to the level in individuals who live and work in the sun and exhibit the lowest risk of MS, it was estimated that an adult who is not exposed to sunlight would need to ingest 4,000 IU/day [87]. This estimate is between the 3,800 IU/day that Goldberg calculated might prevent MS and the 5,000 IU/day that was given in the small clinical trial of fish oil [9, 26]. Important new guidance on vitamin D intakes and serum 25-(OH)-D$_3$ levels was reported recently [93]. Subjects ingesting 1,000 IU/day attained 69 nmole/l serum 25-(OH)-D$_3$ (range 40-100 nmol/l), those ingesting 4,000 IU/day had 96 nmol/l of serum 25-(OH)-D$_3$ (range 69-125 nmol/l), whereas controls taking no supplements had 47 nmol/l. Clearly, an intake far greater than the currently recommended intakes will be required to test the benefits of vitamin D supplementation in MS.

Very high doses of vitamin D can cause hypercalcemia, which is potentially fatal. Accordingly, a tolerable safe upper limit for vitamin D supplementation has been set at 2,000 IU/day for age ≥1 year [88]. However, the panel that established this limit overlooked information indicating that the safe upper limit is actually much higher. Adults living or working in sunny environments easily generate >10,000 IU/day of vitamin D through sun exposure without adverse effects, so the safe upper limit for total vitamin D nutrition is at least 10,000 IU/day [87]. All documented cases of vitamin D toxicity with hypercalcemia involved intakes ≥40,000 IU/day [87]. Finally, 4,000 IU/day resulted in serum 25-(OH)-D$_3$ levels that were within the normal range, and no adverse effects were seen [93]. Hence, the current tolerable safe upper limit for vitamin D supplementation will have to yield to the experimental results, moving upward and allowing supplementation in the 1,000-4,000 IU range to be tested for immune system benefits in sunlight-deprived individuals.

To contribute to the well-being of MS patients, and to the growing body of information, it is very important to monitor 25-(OH)-D$_3$ levels and bone health in MS patients, since many of these patients show deficient serum 25-(OH)-D$_3$ levels, reduced bone mass, high bone mass loss rates, and high fracture rates compared with controls [28, 29]. The analysis should be performed 1-2 months after the nadir of solar radiation, and should include measurements of serum 25-(OH)-D$_3$, bone mass, bone turnover, and MS disease activity. The effects on bone health and disease status of supplementation with calcium and vitamin D need to be examined in well-controlled studies. In closing, it is noteworthy that MS and rickets show very similar geographies [94]. In 1822, the geography of rickets led Sniadecki to suggest that sunlight might cure rickets [13]. Regrettably, rickets continued to cripple children for a full century before the benefits of sunlight and cod liver oil were proven, and cod liver oil became a winter staple for children living in northerly latitudes [95, 96]. The evidence linking sunlight, vitamin D, and MS is diverse and robust. It is time to put the hypothesis that vitamin D may be a natural inhibitor of MS to the test.

Acknowledgements. I wish to thank Faye Nashold, Joan Goverman, David Miller, George Ebers, Ashton Embry, Reinhold Vieth, Ian Duncan, Bill Woodward, Fabienne Van de Keere, and Susumu Tonegawa who have contributed greatly to this work. I am indebted to the National Multiple Sclerosis Society grant RG3107-A-2 and the Metropolitan Women's Club of Madison, Wis., for supporting this research.

References

1. Willer CJ, Ebers, GC (2000) Susceptibility to multiple sclerosis: interplay between genes and environment. Curr Opin Neurol 13:241-247
2. Ebers GC, Dyment DA (1998) Genetics of multiple sclerosis. Semin Neurol 18:295-299
3. Ebers GC, Bulman DE, Sadovnick AD et al (1986) A population-based study of multiple sclerosis in twins. N Engl J Med 315:1638-1642
4. Acheson ED, Bachrach CA, Wright FM (1960) Some comments on the relationship of the distribution of multiple sclerosis to latitude, solar radiation and other variables. Acta Psychiatr Scand 35 [Suppl 147]:132-147
5. Freedman DM, Dosemeci M, Alavanja MC (2000) Mortality from multiple sclerosis and exposure to residential and occupational solar radiation: a case-control study based on death certificates. Occup Environ Med 57:418-421
6. Kurtzke JF, Kurland LT, Goldberg ID (1971) Mortality and migration in multiple sclerosis. Neurology 21:1186-1197
7. Ebers GC, Sadovnick AD (1994) The role of genetic factors in multiple sclerosis susceptibility. J Neuroimmunol 54:1-17
8. Hammond SR, English DR, McLeod JG (2000) The age-range of risk of developing multiple sclerosis: evidence from a migrant population in Australia. Brain 123:968-974

9. Goldberg P (1974) Multiple sclerosis: vitamin D and calcium as environmental determinants of prevalance (a viewpoint). 1. Sunlight, dietary factors and epidemiology. Int J Environ Studies 6:19-27

10. Hayes CE, Cantorna MT, De Luca HF (1997) Vitamin D and multiple sclerosis. Proc Soc Exp Biol Med 216:21-27

11. Hayes CE (2000) Vitamin D: a natural inhibitor of multiple sclerosis. Proc Nutr Soc 59:531-535

12. Fuller KE, Casparian JM (2001) Vitamin D: balancing cutaneous and systemic considerations. South Med J 94:58-64

13. Holick MF (1995) Environmental factors that influence the cutaneous production of vitamin D. Am J Clin Nutr 61:638S-645S

14. Velluz L, Amiard G (1949) Chimie organique-equilibre de reaction entre precalciferol et calciferol. Comptes Rendus de l'Academie des Sciences 228:853

15. Holick M, Schnoes HK, De Luca HF (1971) Identification of 1,25-dihydroxycholecalciferol, a form of vitamin D3 metabolically active in the intestine. Proc Natl Acad Sci U S A 68:803-804

16. Norman AW, Myrtle JF, Midgett RJ, Nowicki HG, Williams V, Popjak G (1971) 1,25-Dihydroxycholecalciferol: identification of the proposed active form of vitamin D3 in the intestine. Science 173:51-54

17. Webb AR, Kline L, Holick MF (1988) Influence of season and latitude on the cutaneous synthesis of vitamin D3: exposure to winter sunlight in Boston and Edmonton will not promote vitamin D3 synthesis in human skin. J Clin Endocrinol Metab 67:373-378

18. Haussler MR, Haussler CA, Jurutka PW, Thompson PD, Hsieh JC, Remus LS, Selznick SH, Whitfield GK (1998) The vitamin D hormone and its nuclear receptor: molecular actions and disease states. J Endocrinol 154 [Suppl]:S57-S73

19. Jones G, Strugnell SA, De Luca HF (1998) Current understanding of the molecular actions of vitamin D. Physiol Rev 78:1193-1231

20. Steckley JL, Dyment DA, Sadovnick AD, Risch N, Hayes C, Ebers GC (2000) Genetic analysis of vitamin D related genes in Canadian multiple sclerosis patients. Canadian Collaborative Study Group. Neurology 54:729-732

21. Arnason A, Jensson O, Skaftadottir I, Birgisdottir B, Gudmundsson G, Johannesson G (1980) HLA types, GC protein and other genetic markers in multiple sclerosis and two other neurological diseases in Iceland. Acta Neurol Scand 62 [Suppl 78]:39-40

22. Fukazawa T, Yabe I, Kikuchi S, Sasaki H, Hamada T, Miyasaka K, Tashiro K (1999) Association of vitamin D receptor gene polymorphism with multiple sclerosis in Japanese. J Neurol Sci 166:47-52

23. Niino M, Fukazawa T, Yabe I, Kikuchi S, Sasaki H, Tashiro K (2000) Vitamin D receptor gene polymorphism in multiple sclerosis and the association with HLA class II alleles. J Neurol Sci 177:65-71

24. Nashold FE, Hoag KA, Goverman J, Hayes CE (2001) Rag-1-dependent cells are necessary for 1,25-dihydroxyvitamin D3 prevention of experimental autoimmune encephalomyelitis. J Neuroimmunol 119:16-29

25. Swank RL, Lerstad O, Strom A, Backer J (1952) Multiple sclerosis in rural Norway: its geographic and occupational incidence in relation to nutrition. N Engl J Med 246:721-728

26. Goldberg P, Fleming MC, Picard EH (1986) Multiple sclerosis: decreased relapse rate through dietary supplementation with calcium, magnesium and vitamin D. Med Hypotheses 21:193-200

27. Nordvik I, Myhr KM, Nyland H, Bjerve KS (2000) Effect of dietary advice and n-3 supplementation in newly diagnosed MS patients. Acta Neurol Scand 102:143-149

28. Nieves J, Cosman F, Herbert J, Shen V, Lindsay R (1994) High prevalence of vitamin D deficiency and reduced bone mass in multiple sclerosis. Neurology 44:1687-1692

29. Cosman F, Nieves J, Komar L, Ferrer G, Herbert J, Formica C, Shen V, Lindsay R (1998) Fracture history and bone loss in patients with MS. Neurology 51:1161-1165

30. Wuthrich R, Rieder HP (1970) The seasonal incidence of multiple sclerosis in Switzerland. Eur Neurol 3:257-264

31. Bamford CR, Sibley WA, Thies C (1983) Seasonal variation of multiple sclerosis exacerbations in Arizona. Neurology 33:697-701

32. Goodkin DE, Hertsgaard D (1989) Seasonal variation of multiple sclerosis exacerbations in North Dakota. Arch Neurol 46:1015-1018

33. Jin YP, de Pedro-Cuesta J, Soderstrom M, Link H (1999) Incidence of optic neuritis in Stockholm, Sweden, 1990-1995: II. Time and space patterns. Arch Neurol 56:975-980

34. Auer DP, Schumann EM, Kumpfel T, Gossl C, Trenkwalder C (2000) Seasonal fluctuations of gadolinium-enhancing magnetic resonance imaging lesions in multiple sclerosis. Ann Neurol 47:276-277

35. Embry AF, Snowdon LR, Vieth R (2000) Vitamin D and seasonal fluctuations of gadolinium-enhancing magnetic resonance imaging lesions in multiple sclerosis. Ann Neurol 48:271-272

36. Olitsky PK, Yager RH (1949) Experimental disseminated encephalomyelitis in white mice. J Exp Med 90:213

37. Cantorna MT, Hayes CE, De Luca HF (1996) 1,25-Dihydroxyvitamin D3 reversibly blocks the progression of relapsing encephalomyelitis, a model of multiple sclerosis. Proc Natl Acad Sci U S A 93:7861-7864

38. Cantorna MT, Humpal-Winter J, De Luca HF (1999) Dietary calcium is a major factor in 1,25-dihydroxycholecalciferol suppression of experimental autoimmune encephalomyelitis in mice. J Nutr 129:1966-1971

39. Lemire JM, Archer DC (1991) 1,25-dihydroxyvitamin D3 prevents the in vivo induction of murine experimental autoimmune encephalomyelitis. J Clin Invest 87:1103-1107

40. Nashold FE, Miller DJ, Hayes CE (2000) 1,25-dihydroxyvitamin D3 treatment decreases macrophage accumulation in the CNS of mice with experimental autoimmune encephalomyelitis. J Neuroimmunol 103:171-179

41. Bhalla AK, Amento EP, Clemens TL, Holick MF, Krane SM (1983) Specific high-affinity receptors for 1,25-dihydroxyvitamin D3 in human peripheral blood mononuclear cells: presence in monocytes and induction in T lymphocytes following activation. J Clin Endocrinol Metab 57:1308-1310

42. Provvedini DM, Tsoukas CD, Deftos LJ, Manolagas SC (1983) 1,25-dihydroxyvitamin D3 receptors in human leukocytes. Science 221:1181-1183

43. Veldman CM, Cantorna, MT, De Luca HF (2000) Expression of 1,25-dihydroxyvitamin D(3) receptor in the immune system. Arch Biochem Biophys 374:334-338

44. Reichel H, Koeffler HP, Tobler A, Norman AW (1987) 1 alpha,25-Dihydroxyvitamin D3 inhibits gamma-interferon synthesis by normal human peripheral blood lymphocytes. Proc Natl Acad Sci U S A 84:3385-3389

45. Rigby WF, Denome S, Fanger MW (1987) Regulation of lymphokine production and human T lymphocyte activation by 1,25-dihydroxyvitamin D3. Specific inhibition at the level of messenger RNA. J Clin Invest 79:1659-1664

46. Rigby WF (1988) The immunobiology of vitamin D. Immunol Today 9:54-58

47. Lemire JM, Archer DC, Beck L, Spiegelberg HL (1995) Immunosuppressive actions of 1,25-dihydroxyvitamin D3: preferential inhibition of Th1 functions. J Nutr 125:1704S-1708S

48. Muller K, Bendtzen K (1996) 1,25-Dihydroxyvitamin D3 as a natural regulator of human immune functions. J Invest Dermatol Symp Proc 1:68-71

49. Lemire J (2000) 1,25-Dihydroxyvitamin D3--a hormone with immunomodulatory properties. Z Rheumatol 59:24-27

50. D'Ambrosio D, Cippitelli M, Cocciolo MG, Mazzeo D, Di Lucia P, Lang R, Sinigaglia F, Panina-Bordignon P (1998) Inhibition of IL-12 production by 1,25-dihydroxyvit-

amin D3. Involvement of NF-kappaB downregulation in transcriptional repression of the p40 gene. J Clin Invest 101:252-262

51. Griffin MD, Lutz WH, Phan VA, Bachman LA, McKean DJ, Kumar R (2000) Potent inhibition of dendritic cell differentiation and maturation by vitamin D analogs. Biochem Biophys Res Commun 270:701-708

52. Penna G, Adorini L (2000) 1 Alpha,25-dihydroxyvitamin D3 inhibits differentiation, maturation, activation, and survival of dendritic cells leading to impaired alloreactive T cell activation. J Immunol 164:2405-2411

53. Piemonti L, Monti P, Sironi M, Fraticelli P, Leone BE, Dal Cin E, Allavena P, Di Carlo V (2000) Vitamin D3 affects differentiation, maturation, and function of human monocyte-derived dendritic cells. J Immunol 164:4443-4451

54. Trinchieri G, Scott P (1999) Interleukin-12: basic principles and clinical applications. Curr Top Microbiol Immunol 238:57-78

55. Zamvil SS, Mitchell DJ, Moore AC, Kitamura K, Steinman L, Rothbard JB (1986) T-cell epitope of the autoantigen myelin basic protein that induces encephalomyelitis. Nature 324:258-260

56. Goverman J, Woods A, Larson L, Weiner LP, Hood L, Zaller DM (1993) Transgenic mice that express a myelin basic protein-specific T cell receptor develop spontaneous autoimmunity. Cell 72:551-560

57. Cantorna MT, Woodward WD, Hayes CE, De Luca HF (1998) 1,25-dihydroxyvitamin D3 is a positive regulator for the two anti- encephalitogenic cytokines TGF-beta 1 and IL-4. J Immunol 160:5314-5319

58. Cantorna MT, Humpal-Winter J, De Luca HF (2000) In vivo upregulation of interleukin-4 is one mechanism underlying the immunoregulatory effects of 1,25-dihydroxyvitamin D(3). Arch Biochem Biophys 377:135-138

59. Van de Keere F, Tonegawa S (1998) CD4(+) T cells prevent spontaneous experimental autoimmune encephalomyelitis in anti-myelin basic protein T cell receptor transgenic mice. J Exp Med 188:1875-1882

60. Olivares-Villagomez D, Wang Y, Lafaille JJ (1998) Regulatory CD4(+) T cells expressing endogenous T cell receptor chains protect myelin basic protein-specific transgenic mice from spontaneous autoimmune encephalomyelitis. J Exp Med 188:1883-1894

61. Brabb T, von Dassow P, Ordonez N, Schnabel B, Duke B, Goverman J (2000) In situ tolerance within the central nervous system as a mechanism for preventing autoimmunity. J Exp Med 192:871-880

62. Pyke DA (1969) The geography of diabetes. Postgrad Med J [Suppl]:796-801

63. Group DERI (1988) Geographic patterns of childhood insulin-dependent diabetes mellitus. Diabetes 37:1113-1119

64. Green A, Gale EA, Patterson CC et al (1992) Incidence of childhood-onset insulin-dependent diabetes mellitus: the EURODIAB ACE Study. Lancet 339:905-909

65. Nystrom L, Dahlquist G, Ostman J, Wall S, Arnqvist H, Blohme G, Lithner F, Littorin B, Schersten B, Wibell L (1992) Risk of developing insulin-dependent diabetes mellitus (IDDM) before 35 years of age: indications of climatological determinants for age at onset. Int J Epidemiol 21:352-358

66. Williams DR (1993) Epidemiological and geographic factors in diabetes. Eye 7:202-204

67. Dahlquist G, Mustonen L (1994) Childhood onset diabetes--time trends and climatological factors. Int J Epidemiol 23:1234-1241

68. McDermott MF, Ramachandran A, Ogunkolade BW, Aganna E, Curtis D, Boucher BJ, Snehalatha C, Hitman GA (1997) Allelic variation in the vitamin D receptor influences susceptibility to IDDM in Indian Asians. Diabetologia 40:971-975

69. Group ES (1999) Vitamin D supplement in early childhood and risk for type I (insulin-dependent) diabetes mellitus. Diabetologia 42:51-54

70. Mathieu C, Waer M, Laureys J, Rutgeerts O, Bouillon R (1994) Prevention of autoimmune diabetes in NOD mice by 1,25 dihydroxyvitamin D3. Diabetologia 37:552-558

71. Sonnenberg A, McCarty DJ, Jacobsen SJ (1991) Geographic variation of inflammatory bowel disease within the United States. Gastroenterology 100:143-149
72. Sonnenberg A, Wasserman IH (1991) Epidemiology of inflammatory bowel disease among U.S. military veterans. Gastroenterology 101:122-130
73. Shivananda S, Lennard-Jones J, Logan R, Fear N, Price A, Carpenter L, van Blankenstein M (1996) Incidence of inflammatory bowel disease across Europe: is there a difference between north and south? Results of the European Collaborative Study on Inflammatory Bowel Disease (EC-IBD). Gut 39:690-697
74. Sonnenberg A (1986) Geographic variation in the incidence of and mortality from inflammatory bowel disease. Dis Colon Rectum 29:854-861
75. Sonnenberg, A (1990) Occupational distribution of inflammatory bowel disease among German employees. Gut 31:1037-1040
76. Sonnenberg A (1990) Occupational mortality of inflammatory bowel disease. Digestion 46:10-18
77. Cucino C, Sonnenberg A (2001) Occupational mortality from inflammatory bowel disease in the United States 1991-1996. Am J Gastroenterol 96:1101-1105
78. Aslan A, Triadafilopoulos G (1992) Fish oil fatty acid supplementation in active ulcerative colitis: a double-blind, placebo-controlled, crossover study. Am J Gastroenterol 87:432-437
79. Stenson WF, Cort D, Rodgers J, Burakoff R, De Schryver-Kecskemeti K, Gramlich TL, Beeken W (1992) Dietary supplementation with fish oil in ulcerative colitis. Ann Intern Med 116:609-614
80. O'Sullivan MA, O'Morain CA (1998) Nutritional therapy in Crohn's disease. Inflamm Bowel Dis 4:45-53
81. Fournier C, Gepner P, Sadouk M, Charreire J (1990) In vivo beneficial effects of cyclosporin A and 1,25-dihydroxyvitamin D3 on the induction of experimental autoimmune thyroiditis. Clin Immunol Immunopathol 54:53-63
82. Lemire JM, Ince A, Takashima M (1992) 1,25-Dihydroxyvitamin D3 attenuates the expression of experimental murine lupus of MRL/l mice. Autoimmunity 12:143-148
83. Cantorna MT, Hayes CE, De Luca HF (1998) 1,25-Dihydroxycholecalciferol inhibits the progression of arthritis in murine models of human arthritis. J Nutr 128:68-72
84. Holick MF (2001) Sunlight "D"ilemma: risk of skin cancer or bone disease and muscle weakness. Lancet 357:4-6
85. Malabanan A, Veronikis IE, Holick MF (1998) Redefining vitamin D insufficiency. Lancet 351:805-806
86. Chapuy MC, Preziosi P, Maamer M, Arnaud S, Galan P, Hercberg S, Meunier PJ (1997) Prevalence of vitamin D insufficiency in an adult normal population. Osteoporos Int 7:439-443
87. Vieth R (1999) Vitamin D supplementation, 25-hydroxyvitamin D concentrations, and safety. Am J Clin Nutr 69:842-856
88. Holick MF (1998) Vitamin D requirements for humans of all ages: new increased requirements for women and men 50 years and older. Osteoporos Int 8:S24-S29
89. Utiger RD (1998) The need for more vitamin D. N Engl J Med 338:828-829
90. Glerup H, Mikkelsen K, Poulsen L, Hass E, Overbeck S, Thomsen J, Charles P, Eriksen EF (2000) Commonly recommended daily intake of vitamin D is not sufficient if sunlight exposure is limited. J Intern Med 247:260-268
91. Zerath E, Holy X, Gaud R, Schmitt D (1999) Decreased serum levels of 1,25-(OH)2 vitamin D during 1 year of sunlight deprivation in the Antarctic. Eur J Appl Physiol Occup Physiol 79:141-147
92. Compston JE (1998) Vitamin D deficiency: time for action. Evidence supports routine supplementation for elderly people and others at risk. BMJ 317:1466-1467
93. Vieth R, Chan PC, MacFarlane GD (2001) Efficacy and safety of vitamin D(3) intake exceeding the lowest observed adverse effect level. Am J Clin Nutr 73:288-294

94. Hess AF, Unger LF (1929) Rickets, osteomalacia and tetany. Lea and Febiger, Philadelphia, pp 38-61
95. Hess AF, Unger LF (1921) Cure of infantile rickets by sunlight. JAMA 39:77-82
96. Chick H, Dalyell EJ, Hume M, Mackay HMM, Smith HH (1922) The etiology of rickets in infants: prophylactic and curative observations at the Vienna University Kinderklinik. Lancet 1:7-12

Chapter 19

The Yin and Yang of Inflammation in Multiple Sclerosis

G. Giovannoni

Introduction

Multiple sclerosis (MS) is a clinically heterogeneous disease [1]. On the one side of the spectrum is relapsing-remitting (RR) disease, characterized by attacks of neurological dysfunction due to focal central nervous system (CNS) inflammation, followed by recovery and a period of remission, and on the other side is primary progressive (PP) disease, which is progressive from the outset with no clinical relapses. Between these two extremes are patients who, after presenting with RR disease, subsequently go onto develop a secondary progressive (SP) course. SP disease can be further subdivided into relapsing and non-relapsing disease, depending on whether or not patients continue to have clinical relapses. Approximately 15%-30% of patients with RR disease do not enter the progressive phase of the disease and are classified retrospectively as having benign disease. Why such clinical heterogeneity occurs is currently unknown. Are RR and PPMS different diseases or are they part of the same clinical spectrum? Why do some patients develop progressive disease whilst others do not? Answers to these questions will not only improve our understanding of MS, but will also have major implications for the treatment of MS. Recent data support a complex role for inflammation in disease pathogenesis, with good and bad effects. This article will review the supporting data and propose a hypothesis to explain this paradox or yin and yang of inflammation.

Central Versus Peripheral Compartment

The CNS, like the eye and testes, differs from other organ systems in that it is an immune-privileged site, protected to a lesser or greater degree by various barriers [2]. Systemically administered immunomodulatory or immunosuppressive therapies may therefore not necessarily penetrate into the CNS to have the desired local effects. However, the systemic effects of these therapies may not necessarily be desirable, as several inflammatory mediators have pleiotropic functions, e.g., tumor necrosis factor-α (TNF-α) and nitric oxide (NO), which modulate the immune system.

Anti-TNF Therapies

TNF-α is a pro-inflammatory cytokine pivotal in autoimmune disease and is associated with cell-mediated inflammation. It has been strongly implicated in the pathogenesis of MS [3]. Systemic inhibition of TNF-α activity using either a neutralizing anti-TNF-α antibody or soluble TNF-α receptor fusion protein has proved very successful in inflammatory bowel disease and rheumatoid arthritis [4-7]. Unfortunately, this strategy has not proved successful in MS, and in fact has had the opposite effect, with an increase rather than a decrease in disease activity. Firstly, a small pilot study in which a chimeric neutralizing anti-TNF-a antibody (CA2, Centocor) was administered to MS patients had to be aborted because there was a dramatic increase in disease activity on magnetic resonance imaging (MRI) [8]. Secondly, a large multicenter phase III study of soluble TNF-α receptor-Fc receptor fusion protein was stopped prematurely because of an increase in the number of relapses in the actively treated group compared with patients receiving a placebo [9]. Similar effects have been demonstrated in experimental allergic encephalomyelitis (EAE) [10]. TNF-α knockout mice are less resistant to the induction of EAE and develop severe non-remitting disease [10]. The systemic administration of TNF-α induces remission in these animals, whereas the intrathecal administration of TNF-α exacerbates disease [11]. It therefore appears that TNF-α production within the CNS is deleterious, whereas systemic production is immunomodulatory and has a role in inducing remission (Fig. 1).

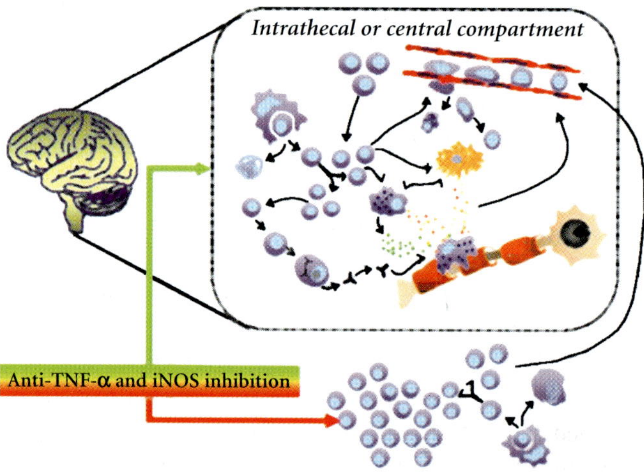

Fig. 1. The double-edged sword of pro-inflammatory mediators. Inhibition of intrathecal tumor necrosis factor-α (TNF-α) activity or inducible nitric oxide production is beneficial in experimental allergic encephalomyelitis (EAE). However, peripheral inhibition of their activity results in a lowering of disease susceptibility and a progressive non-remitting EAE course. Inhibiting peripheral TNF-α activity in patients with multiple sclerosis (MS) results in an increase in magnetic resonance imaging (MRI) activity and more-frequent relapses

Inducible NO

NO plays a role in the pathogenesis of MS [12]. Increased astrocytic NO synthase (NOS) activity and NOS mRNA have been demonstrated in demyelinating lesions [13, 14]. Increased protein nitrosylation [15] and DNA damage [16], the footprints of NO and its reactive product peroxynitrite, have also been shown in MS lesions. Nitrate and nitrite (NO_x), the stable degradation products of NO, are significantly increased in the cerebrospinal fluid (CSF) [17] and serum of MS patients [18]. Interestingly the levels of NO_x are higher in the serum of patients with RR compared with patients with SP disease [19]. In a large cross-sectional study, urinary excretion of NO_x in patients with benign and early RR disease was significantly higher than in patients with progressive disease [20]. These findings, although preliminary, suggest that decreased NO production may be associated with progressive disease. Possible support for this hypothesis comes from recent studies in EAE. In an early study, the NOS2 inhibitor aminoguanidine ameliorated MBP-specific T cell adoptive transfer of EAE in SJL/J mice [21]. However, studies in the Lewis rat have shown that NOS2 inhibitors result in a worsening of the disease course [22, 23]. In addition, it is easier to induce EAE in NOS2 knockout (NOS2-KO) mice than wild-type control mice, and the NOS2 knockout mice have more-severe disease than wild-type control mice [24, 25]. The differences between NOS2-KO and wild-type mice result from a failure of the disease to remit in the NOS2-KO mice. The wild-type mice have a striking ability to recover from EAE compared with NOS2-KO mice. However, inhibiting NOS2 activity within the CNS by the administration of intrathecal antisense oligonucleotides ameliorated EAE [26]. It therefore appears that intrathecal NOS2-induced NO production is deleterious and systemic NO production may have a role in switching off or inducing remission in EAE and possibly MS (Fig. 1).

There is evidence that NO has immunological effects that favorably affect the course of autoimmune disease, which are significant in the context of the above observations in MS and EAE. NO inhibits lymphocyte proliferation and upregulates Th2 cell function, by suppressing interleukin (IL)-2 gene transcription [27] and upregulating IL-4 production [28]. In macrophages, NO induces transcription of the IL-12 $(p40)_2$ homodimer, an antagonist of IL-12 [29], which may further decrease Th1 T cell reactivity. NO decreases macrophage MHC class II expression [30], increases prostaglandin E_2 production [31], and downregulates adhesion molecule expression [32, 33] – effects that are all potentially favorable in autoimmune inflammatory reactions. NO also modulates apoptosis and may play an important role in terminating autoimmune inflammatory reactions by eliminating autoreactive T cells [34].

The effects of TNF-α and NO in EAE and MS are similar and may involve a common pathway. NO has been shown to modulate TNF-α signaling via NF-κB [35], a pivotal second messenger of TNF-α [36], which is redox sensitive. As NO modulates the redox state of a cell, depending on its concentration [37], it is plausible that the effects of TNF-α and NO are mediated via NF-κB.

Trophic Effects of Inflammation

The new insights regarding the beneficial local effects of inflammation are emerging and challenging the rationale of generalized immunosuppression in MS. Inflammation appears to play a role in promoting tissue repair and remyelination via the production of growth or trophic factors that act on oligodendrocyte precursors, oligodendrocytes, and neurones. Brain-derived neurotrophic factor (BDNF) and insulin-like growth factors, which are survival factors for oligodendrocytes [38, 39], and their receptors are upregulated in MS plaques [40, 41]. The three receptors of glial growth factor 2 (GGF2), a neuronal signal that promotes the proliferation and survival of the oligodendrocyte, are found on oligodendrocytes, with increased expression in MS lesions [42]. These observations may explain the apparent failure of generalized immunosuppressive therapies, which would switch off these favorable aspects of inflammation. For example, progressive axonal loss in patients with non-relapsing progressive disease may be due to the withdrawal of trophic support rather than ongoing inflammation. It is widely accepted that MS is an organ-specific autoimmune disease mediated by antigen-specific auto-aggressive T cells. However, it has recently been shown that autoimmunity is not necessarily all bad, and may be beneficial in diseases of the CNS characterized by axonal transection [43].

This yin and yang of inflammation between the central and systemic compartments and the good and bad mediators has important therapeutic implications, and suggests that more-rational or targeted therapeutic approaches should be adopted in MS.

Mechanisms of Disease Progression

The mechanisms underlying disease progression are unknown. Current proposals include failure of reparative and neuroprotective mechanisms, an imbalance between the Th1 and Th2 cell-mediated immune responses, dysregulated T cell function, reduced T cell apoptosis, antigen determinant spreading, pathological heterogeneity, which includes an oligodendrogliopathy and several inflammatory variants [44], and genetic differences responsible for tissue repair and/or protection against tissue damage [45]. Several groups have reported weak associations between genetic polymorphisms in immune response genes and clinical course. Similarly, numerous studies have reported immunological differences between patients with non-progressive and progressive disease. Further studies are required to confirm and to assess the importance of these results. The role inflammation plays in disease progression is not well defined. Although the frequency of clinical attacks early in the course of MS correlates with the later development of disability, MRI and immunological markers of active inflammation are less predictive. Patients with PPMS by definition have no clinical relapses and have little if any MRI activity, but continue to develop progressive disability. We also observed cases with progressive cerebral atrophy (which correlates with the development of neurological impairment [46]), with and without superimposed inflammatory activity measured using gadolinium (Gd)-enhanced MRI and a panel of immunological markers. In addition, immunosuppressive therapies, which are capable of reducing or stopping clinical relapses and suppressing MRI activity, do not necessarily stop disease progression [47].

A Primary Neurodegenerative Hypothesis

MS is primarily a neurodegenerative disease characterized by progressive neuroaxonal loss (Fig. 2). This neuroaxonal loss does not necessarily occur contin-

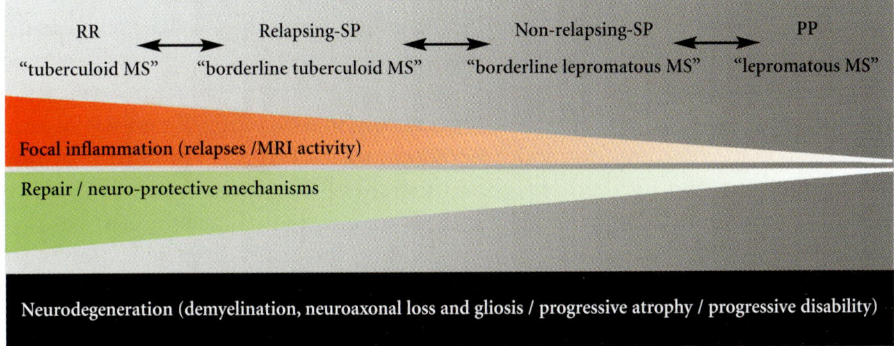

Fig. 2. A primary neurodegenerative hypothesis. Although MS is a clinically heterogeneous disease, it can be viewed as an inflammatory neurodegenerative disease with the clinical spectrum or phenotype determined by the presence or absence of focal inflammation, similar to that which occurs in infectious diseases, e.g., leprosy. The underlying neurodegenerative component of the disease may or may not be ongoing but it is modified by superimposed focal inflammatory events. The focal inflammation may be an appropriate host response directed at an unidentified etiological agent or an inappropriate autoimmune response. These focal inflammatory events are responsible for clinical attacks and MRI disease activity. Although damaging in themselves, the focal inflammation provides the biological substrate in the form of trophic and growth factors, which promote repair and clinical recovery. Inhibiting the focal inflammatory events, e.g., with generalized immunosuppression, would reduce the relapse rate and MRI activity and remove the important trophic and growth factor support provided by the inflammatory infiltrates, but it may not affect the underlying primary neurodegenerative processes. This strategy would simply convert relapsing-remitting (RR) disease into non-relapsing progressive disease. There is evidence from infectious diseases that this phenotypic variability is linked to genetic susceptibility (*SP* secondary progressive, *PP* primary progressive)

uously or at a constant rate. Superimposed focal inflammation, which is responsible for the acute clinical attacks or MRI activity in the form of new or enlarging lesions on T2-weighted MRI or Gd-enhancing lesions on T1-weighted MRI, modifies the clinical course. Although damaging in itself, the focal inflammation supplies important growth and trophic factors to promote recovery. Removing the trophic support may expose the underlying neurodegenerative disease, by converting a relapsing course into a non-relapsing progressive course. Some immunosuppressive therapies appear to have this effect, e.g., CAMPATH-1h or anti-CD52 [47] and cladribine (unpublished data) are very effective in suppressing clinical relapses and MRI activity, but are not effective in preventing disease progression. A corollary to this hypothesis is that the inflammation is an appropriate host response to whatever is causing MS. Removing inflammation simply exposes the underlying primary neurodegenerative disease process.

The phenotypic spectrum observed in patients with MS is not unique to MS, and is also seen in patients with other autoimmune diseases, for example rheumatoid arthritis. Patients with rheumatoid arthritis usually have relapsing-remitting disease early in their disease course, which is supplanted by a chronic progressive phase later in the disease [48]. In addition, small groups of patients with rheumatoid arthritis also have primary progressive and benign disease. The clinical variability in patients with MS and other autoimmune diseases is reminiscent of that which occurs in chronic infection, leprosy being the prototype with the lepromatous and tuberculoid forms representing the polar extremes. I propose that a similar phenomenon is occurring in MS, with PP and RR disease representing the lepromatous and tuberculoid forms respectively, with relapsing SP disease representing the borderline tuberculoid form and non-relapsing SP disease the borderline lepromatous form. As in leprosy this heterogeneity or disease spectrum may influenced by host factors, for example genetic polymorphisms, which control the immune response or the host tissue response to inflammation and injury [49].

Conclusions

In conclusion, MS is an inflammatory neurodegenerative disease. The role inflammation plays in the disease process is complex. On the one hand it causes demyelination and axonal damage and on the other hand it provides growth and trophic factors that promote remyelination and axonal recovery. In addition, the mediators of inflammation have pleiotropic effects, depending on their site of action. Locally produced factors, which are toxic and damaging to oligodendrocytes and axons, may have immunomodulatory effects systemically. Generalized immunosuppression may remove the local trophic support provided by inflammation, exposing the underlying neurodegenerative processes. Poorly targeted therapies may interfere with systemic immunomodulatory processes, which result in unchecked autoimmunity, and fail to reach their desired targets within the CNS, because of poor accessibility due to the blood-brain barrier. We need to reassess our therapeutic strategies in MS in view of the above observations.

References

1. Lublin FD et al (1996) Defining the clinical course of multiple sclerosis: results of an international survey. National Multiple Sclerosis Society (USA) Advisory Committee on Clinical Trials of New Agents in Multiple Sclerosis. Neurology 46:907-911
2. Cserr HF et al (1992) Cervical lymphatics, the blood-brain barrier and the immunoreactivity of the brain: a new view. Immunol Today 13:507-512
3. Raine CS (1995) Multiple sclerosis: TNF revisited, with promise. Nat Med 1:211-214
4. Maini R et al (1999) Infliximab (chimeric anti-tumour necrosis factor alpha monoclonal antibody) versus placebo in rheumatoid arthritis patients receiving concomitant methotrexate: a randomised phase III trial. ATTRACT Study Group. Lancet 354:1932-1939
5. Moreland LW et al (1997) Treatment of rheumatoid arthritis with a recombinant human tumor necrosis factor receptor (p75)-Fc fusion protein. N Engl J Med 337:141-147
6. Hodgson H (1999) Prospects of new therapeutic approaches for Crohn's disease. Lancet 353:425-426
7. Rutgeerts et al (1999) Efficacy and safety of retreatment with anti-tumor necrosis factor antibody (infliximab) to maintain remission in Crohn's disease. Gastroenterology 117:761-769
8. van Oosten BW (1996) Increased MRI activity and immune activation in two multiple sclerosis patients treated with the monoclonal anti-tumor necrosis factor antibody cA2. Neurology 47:1531-1534
9. The Lenercept Multiple Sclerosis Study Group and The University of British Columbia MS/MRI Analysis Group (1999) TNF neutralization in MS: results of a randomized, placebo-controlled multicenter study. Neurology 53:457-465
10. Liu J et al (1998) TNF is a potent anti-inflammatory cytokine in autoimmune-mediated demyelination. Nat Med 4:78-83
11. Dal Canto RA et al (1999) Local delivery of TNF by retrovirus-transduced T lymphocytes exacerbates experimental autoimmune encephalomyelitis. Clin Immunol 90:10-14
12. Giovannoni G et al (1998) The potential role of nitric oxide in multiple sclerosis. Mult Scler 4:212-216
13. Bagasara O et al (1995) Activation of the inducible form of nitric oxide synthase in the brains of patients with multiple sclerosis. Proc Natl Acad Sci U S A 92:12041-12045
14. Bö L et al (1994) Induction of nitric oxide synthase in demyelinating regions of multiple sclerosis brains. Ann Neurol 36:778-786
15. Cross AH et al (1998) Peroxynitrite formation within the central nervous system in active multiple sclerosis. J Neuroimmunol 88:45-56
16. Vladimirova O et al (1998) Oxidative damage to DNA in plaques of MS brains. Mult Scler 4:413-418
17. Johnson AW et al (1995) Evidence for increased nitric oxide production in multiple sclerosis. J Neurol Neurosurg Psychiatry 58:107
18. Giovannoni G et al (1997) Raised serum nitrate and nitrite levels in patients with multiple sclerosis. J Neurol Sci 145:77-81

19. Giovannoni G et al (1997) Raised serum nitrate and nitrite concentrations in patients with multiple sclerosis correlate with lower clinical and MRI levels of disease activity. J Neuroimmunol 80:182

20. Giovannoni G et al (1999) Increased urinary nitric oxide metabolites in patients with multiple sclerosis correlates with early and relapsing disease. Mult Scler 5:335-341

21. Cross AH et al (1994) Aminoguanidine, an inhibitor of inducible nitric oxide synthase, ameliorates experimental autoimmune encephalomyelitis in SJL mice. J Clin Invest 93:2684-2690

22. Zielasek J et al (1995) Administration of nitric oxide synthase inhibitors in experimental autoimmune neuritis and experimental autoimmune encephalomyelitis. J Neuroimmunol 58:81-88

23. Ruuls SR et al (1996) Aggravation of experimental allergic encephalomyelitis (EAE) by administration of nitric oxide (NO) synthase inhibitors. Clin Exp Immunol 103:467-474

24. Fenyk-Melody JE et al (1998) Experimental autoimmune encephalomyelitis is exacerbated in mice lacking the NOS2 gene. J Immunol 160:2940-2946

25. Sahrbacher UC et al (1998) Mice with an inactivation of the inducible nitric oxide synthase gene are susceptible to experimental autoimmune encephalomyelitis. Eur J Immunol 28:1332-1338

26. Ding M et al (1998) Antisense knockdown of inducible nitric oxide synthase inhibits induction of experimental autoimmune encephalomyelitis in SJL/J mice. J Immunol 160:2560-2564

27. Kolb H et al (1998) Nitric oxide in autoimmune disease: cytotoxic or regulatory mediator? Immunol Today 19:556-561

28. Chang RH et al (1997) Nitric oxide increased interleukin-4 expression in T lymphocytes. Immunology 90:364-369

29. Mattner F et al (1993) The interleukin-12 subunit P40 specifically inhibits effects of the interleukin-12 heterodimer. Eur J Immunol 23:2203-2208

30. Sicher SC et al (1994) Inhibition of macrophage Ia expression by nitric oxide. J Immunol 153:1293-1300

31. Habib A et al (1997) Regulation of the expression of cyclooxygenase-2 by nitric oxide in rat peritoneal macrophages. J Immunol 158:3845-3851

32. Kubes P et al (1991) Nitric oxide – an endogenous modulator of leukocyte adhesion. Proc Natl Acad Sci U S A 88:4651-4655

33. Adams MR et al (1997) L-arginine reduces human monocyte adhesion to vascular endothelium and endothelial expression of cell adhesion molecules. Circulation 95:662-668

34. Okuda Y et al (1997) Nitric oxide via an inducible isoform of nitric oxide synthase is a possible factor to eliminate inflammatory cells from the central nervous system of mice with experimental allergic encephalomyelitis. J Neuroimmunol 73:107-116

35. Nathan C (1995) Inducible nitric oxide synthase: regulation subserves function. Curr Top Microbiol Immunol 196:1-4

36. Wajant H et al (1999) TNF receptor associated factors in cytokine signaling. Cytokine Growth Factor Rev 10:15-26

37. Stefanelli C et al (1999) Nitric oxide can function as either a killer molecule or an antiapoptotic effector in cardiomyocytes. Biochim Biophys Acta 1450:406-413

38. Kerschensteiner M et al (1999) Activated human T cells, B cells, and monocytes produce brain-derived neurotrophic factor in vitro and in inflammatory brain lesions: a neuroprotective role of inflammation? J Exp Med 189:865-870

39. Ye P et al (1999) Insulin-like growth factor I protects oligodendrocytes from tumor necrosis factor-alpha-induced injury. Endocrinology 140:3063-3072

40. Wilczak N et al (1997) Insulin-like growth factor-I receptors in normal appearing white matter and chronic plaques in multiple sclerosis. Brain Res 772:243-246

41. Gveric D et al (1999) Insulin-like growth factors and binding proteins in multiple sclerosis plaques. Neuropathol Appl Neurobiol 25:215-225
42. Cannella B (1999) Neuregulin and erbB receptor expression in normal and diseased human white matter. J Neuroimmunol 100:233-242
43. Cohen IR et al (1999) Autoimmune maintenance and neuroprotection of the central nervous system. J Neuroimmunol 100:111-114
44. Lucchinetti CF et al (1996) Distinct patterns of multiple sclerosis pathology indicates heterogeneity on pathogenesis. Brain Pathol 6:259-274
45. Mann CL et al (2000) Glutathione S-transferase polymorphisms in MS: their relationship to disability. Neurology 54:552-557
46. Losseff NA et al (1996) Progressive cerebral atrophy in multiple sclerosis. A serial MRI study. Brain 119:2009-2019
47. Coles AJ et al (1999) Monoclonal antibody treatment exposes three mechanisms underlying the clinical course of multiple sclerosis. Ann Neurol 46:296-304
48. Eberhardt K et al (1998) Clinical course and remission rate in patients with early rheumatoid arthritis: relationship to outcome after 5 years. Br J Rheumatol 37:1324-1329
49. Levin M et al (1999) Understanding the genetic basis of susceptibility to mycobacterial infection. Proc Assoc Am Physicians 111:308-312

Management of Interferon-β1b (Betaseron) Failures in Multiple Sclerosis with Interferon-αn3 (Alferon N)

W.A. Sheremata, A. Minagar

Introduction

The introduction of interferon-β1b (IFN-β1b, Betaseron) in 1993 heralded a new era in the management of multiple sclerosis (MS). A modest overall reduction of exacerbations of 33.8% was enhanced by a 47% reduction for "moderately severe and severe exacerbations", as defined in the protocol [1]. Adverse experience with IFN-β1b, however, was encountered in the majority of trial participants, as well as in the clinical setting [1, 2].

"Flu-like" symptoms occurred in the majority of IFN-β1b recipients, especially early in treatment, with fever occurring in 58% [1, 2]. Cutaneous reactions, consisting of injection site erythema, occurred in 69%, with cutaneous ulceration in 10% or more [3, 4]. In addition, patients with more-active disease do not regularly respond to treatment and occasionally may be perceived to worsen coincident with treatment. The standards committee of the American Academy of Neurology recommended in 1994 that "if reasonable evidence suggests that the drug *does not* prevent exacerbations, or if disease *progression continues* in spite of the drug, withdrawal should be considered" [2, 5].

We now report the use of interferon-αn3 (IFN-αn3) to replace IFN-β1b in 18 of an original group of 100 where adverse experience necessitated withdrawal of IFN-β1b. To evaluate their response they were matched for sex and age with subjects tolerant to IFN-β1b and followed for at least 2 years.

Patients and Methods

Patient Population

One hundred patients were prospectively placed on IFN-β1b, 8 MIU on alternate days, in the context of a phase IV trial, with recruitment beginning in December 1993. All patients were prospectively evaluated and examined on a 3-monthly basis. Follow-up continued on the same basis following the termination of the planned safety study according to FDA guidelines. Disability was recorded using the Kurtzke extended disability status scale (EDSS) and adverse experience collected. Standard hematology and biochemical profiles were obtained and were repeated on a 3-monthly basis. Eighteen patients experi-

Table 1. Demographics of interferon (IFN)-β1b-intolerant and IFNβ1b-tolerant multiple sclerosis (MS) patients

Patient population	Sex	Mean age (years ± SD)	Mean duration of MS
IFN-β1b intolerant	15 F:3M	29±8	7.6±5.5
IFN-β1b tolerant	15 F:3M	31±10.2	4.6±3.8

enced significant adverse effects that led to discontinuation of IFN-β1b treatment and replacement with IFN-αn3. All had been encouraged to continue treatment with IFN-β1b despite their difficulties for at least 6 months, so as to maximize the likelihood of spontaneous resolution. All patients with ulceration had received IFN-β1b treatment only. These patients with adverse effects were matched for sex and for age±3 years with IFN-β1b-tolerant recipients for purposes of outcome comparison (Table 1). Patients were all of European descent.

IFN-αn3

IFN-αn3 (Alferon, Interferon Sciences, New Brunswick N.J., USA) is a highly pure ($\geq 2 \times 10^8$ IU/mg) affinity purified preparation containing multiple natural human IFN-α subtypes [6]. The product became available in 1993 and contains no IFN-β or IFN-O. Use of IFN-αn3 in human trials has demonstrated it to be remarkably free of injection site reactions and relatively free of systemic reactions. A dose of 5 MIU on alternate days was based on previous trials using "Cantell" standard IFN-αn [7].

Demographics and EDSS of 18 patients (15 women and 3 men) experiencing severe skin reactions and/or progressed rapidly despite IFN-β1b, and who discontinued the drug and were started on IFN-αn3 (group 1), are compared with 18 patients matched for age and sex who tolerated and continued IFN-β1b (group 2) (Table 1).

Results

There were 15 women and 3 men in groups 1 and 2. Table 1 shows age at onset of MS for groups 1 and 2 (29±8 vs. 31±10.2 years), EDSS (4.4 vs 4.6), and duration of illness (7.6±5.5 vs. 4.6±3.8 years). The IFN-β1b-intolerant patients had a longer mean duration of illness. Differences were not statistically significant between the groups for any parameter.

Drug

IFN-β1b was discontinued after a mean of 17±9.8 months and IFN-αn3, at a dose of 5 MIU, was initiated on alternate days (group 1). Reasons for withdrawal of IFN-β1b included severe continuing skin reactions in 14, with ulceration in 6, necrosis without ulceration in 1, intense local reaction without ulceration in 7, and extensive subcutaneous nodule formation in 1. Five patients with cutaneous ulcers had continued exacerbations and increasing disability and 4 with marked local reactions (1 hemorrhagic) progressed despite treatment with IFN-β1b. Five subjects progressed rapidly despite treatment. One woman, a physician, had recurrent high fevers that were incapacitating, as well significant loss of well being.

Disability

Mean EDSS was calculated for each group 1 and 2 years after treatment. Patients improving, stabilizing, or worsening by one EDSS grade are shown (Fig. 1). After 1 year, EDSS in group 1 was decreased or unchanged in 16 (89%) of IFN-αn3-treated patients (decreased in 8, unchanged in 8, and increased in 2). In group 2 where IFN-β1b treatment was continued because of drug tolerance, EDSS was decreased or unchanged in 14 (78%) of the patients (decreased in 5, unchanged in 10, and increased in 3). Although twice as many suffered increased disability with continued IFN-β1b therapy, results were not statistically significant. After 2 years, EDSS in group 1 was decreased or unchanded in 14 (78%) IFN-αn3-treated patients (decreased in 6, unchanged in 8, and increased in 4). In group 2, EDSS was decreased or unchanged in 11 (63%) IFN-β1b-treated patients (decreased in 3, unchanged in 8, and increased in 4).

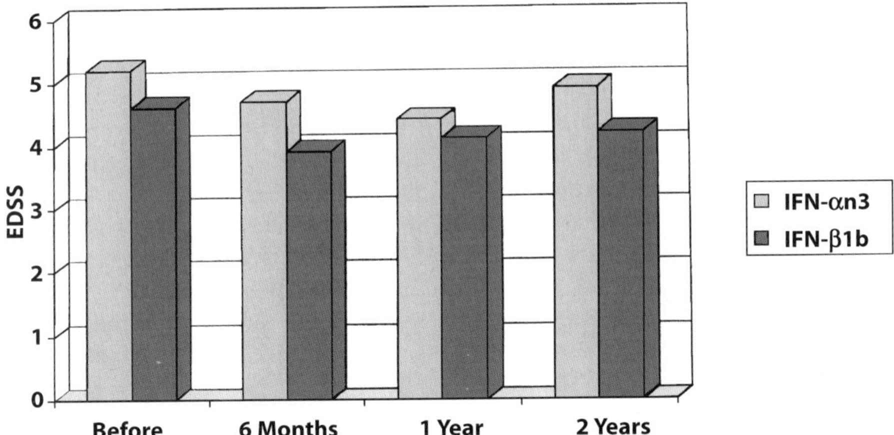

Fig. 1. EDSS of multiple sclerosis patients before and after 6 months, 1 year, and 2 years of interferon (IFN)-αn3 vs IFN-β1b treatment

Adverse Experience

No cutaneous ulceration occurred in group 1 (IFN-αn3-treated), but new cutaneous ulceration occurred in 4 patients in group 2. Two patients suffered multiple ulcers. One patient in group 1 discontinued treatment after the 1st year and deteriorated markedly in the 2nd year. Two other interrupted treatment but continued. One with a history of menorrhagia and anemia experienced a minor degree of thrombocytopenia and stopped IFN-αn3 therapy temporarily, but resumed after a hysterectomy. In group 2, 2 patients interrupted treatment because of adverse experience. A third discontinued treatment because of cutaneous ulceration just after the end of the 2-year follow-up.

We have reviewed magnetic resonance imaging studies from 31 patients on IFN-αn3 including the present group and 38 untreated patients. Gadolinium-enhancing lesions were seen in only 2 (6.5%), whereas 37% of 38 untreated patients were positive [8].

Conclusions

Management of adverse experience encountered with IFN-β1b treatment is a controversial area. Steroids have been advocated to minimize both local and systemic reactions, with limited success and uncertain impact on the course of MS. The successful use of IFN-α as an alternative type I IFN in the management of hairy cell leukemia, as well as observed tolerance of IFN-αn in an earlier dose ranging trial, prompted us to use IFN-αn3 [3]. We employed doses equivalent to those we previously found to be tolerated by MS patients and which stopped intrathecal IgG synthesis [3]. These doses also appeared to prevent exacerbations of MS.

In MS patients intolerant to IFN-β1b, we found IFN-αn3 to be safe and well tolerated. These patients who had experienced severe cutaneous and systemic reactions necessitating withdrawal of IFN-β1b did not experience any local reactions and systemic reactions were minor and generally well tolerated. The observed effect of IFN-αn3 on EDSS in MS was similar to IFN-β1b in patients initially tolerant to IFN-β1b and who continued IFN-β1b treatment. In addition, we found a dramatic reduction in gadolinium-enhancing lesions with IFN-αn3 treatment. IFN-αn3 should be considered in all patients intolerant to IFN-β. Trials of IFN-αn3 as primary treatment of MS are warranted, based on its safety and tolerance.

References

1. The IFNB Multiple Sclerosis Study Group (1993) Interferon beta-1b is effective in relapsing-remitting multiple sclerosis. I. Clinical results of a multicenter, randomized, double-blind, placebo-controlled trial. Neurology 43:655-661

2. Report of the Quality Standards Subcommittee of the AAN (1994) Neurology 44:1537-1540
3. Shcremata WA, Taylor A, Elgart GW (1995) Severe necrotizing cutaneous lesions complicating interferon-beta-1b: clinical features and biopsy results. N Engl J Med 332:23
4. Elgart GW, Sheremata WA, Ahn YS (1997) Cutaneous reactions to recombinant interferon-beta-1b: the clinical and histologic spectrum. J Am Acad Dermatol 37:553-558
5. Paty DW, Hartung HP, Ebers GC et al (1999) Management of relapsing-remitting multiple sclerosis: diagnosis and treatment guidelines. Eur Neurol 6 [Suppl 1]:S1-S35
6. Di Paola M, Ogin E, Smith Y et al (1992) Interferon-a subtypes in natural human leukocyte interferon (interferonα-n3). J Interferon Res 12:S318
7. Squillacote D, Martinez M, Sheremata WA (1996) Natural alpha interferon in multiple sclerosis: preliminary results and follow-up. J Int Med Res 24:246-257
8. Sheremata W, Minagar A, Whiteman M, Onufer J (2001) Interferon-alfa-n3 (Alferon N) reduces gadolinium enhancing brain lesions in multiple sclerosis. J Neurosci 187 [Suppl 1] S454

Subject Index